MW00464779

HEALTHY DAD SICK DAD

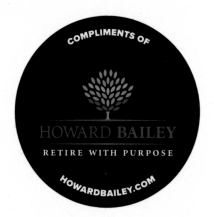

COMPLIMENTS OF

HOWARD BAILEY

RETIRE WITH PURPOSE

HOWARDBAILEY.COM

WHAT GOOD IS YOUR WEALTH
IF YOU DON'T HAVE YOUR HEALTH?

Healthy
DAD

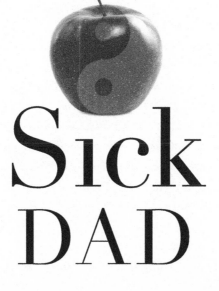

Sick
DAD

DR. GLEN N. ROBISON

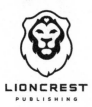

LIONCREST
PUBLISHING

COPYRIGHT © 2021 GLEN N. ROBISON

All rights reserved. "Healthy Dad, Sick Dad" is a common-law trademark (United States Registration pending serial number 88846364) of Live It Lifestyle, LLC. "Rich Dad ®" is a registered trademark of Cash Flow Technologies, Inc. Live It Lifestyle, LLC is NOT IN ANY WAY affiliated with, associated with, endorsed by, or sponsored by Cash Flow Technologies, Inc. nor any subsidiary or affiliate of Cash Flow Technologies, Inc. Live It Lifestyle, LLC is further NOT IN ANY WAY affiliated with, associated with, endorsed by, or sponsored by Robert Kiyosaki.

HEALTHY DAD SICK DAD

What Good Is Your Wealth If You Don't Have Your Health?

ISBN   978-1-5445-2075-9 *Hardcover*
          978-1-5445-2074-2 *Paperback*
          978-1-5445-2073-5 *Ebook*

Contents

—

Introduction

———

What do you get when you live on muffins, root beer floats, and one-dollar tacos while spending 4,000 hours in the classroom and ten years of straight education that cost over $232,000?

Awareness that my personal health crisis was about to happen, and that all the time and money spent in medical school could not offer me the answer to the one question that I was so desperately seeking when I watched my daughter in pain every time she tried to eat over a four-week period. The emergency room visits, the medical tests and the hours spent in the specialty clinics all told me the same thing that I already knew: "There was no answer as to why she had pain when she ate."

What cured my daughter in minutes? It was my Healthy Dad's amazing knowledge and miraculous hands. This opened the floodgates to my questions. It was this experience that left me speechless and became my personal turning point.

Reflecting on all those years in school, I realized not a single class on nutrition was required to become a doctor. So where did I learn all this knowledge? I learned it by observing my biological father (my Sick Dad) who went from being healthy to sick when he approached his retirement years. And I learned it from asking questions to my Healthy Dad who became even more active while remaining healthy when he retired.

Most diets have one goal in mind: to lose weight. Losing weight does not always equate to being healthy just as having a bowel movement does not always equate to eliminating all those toxins out of your body. So why not lose the weight, strengthen your immune system, and have better health all at the same time? This book aims to help you with that! It is a commonsense approach to your health.

My goal for those who read this book is primarily to get you to start **ASKING** questions about your own health. Second, I want to help you understand that you cannot remedy a lifestyle that relies on remedies and fad diets. And last, explain that in nature when you are balanced, there are no diseases.

WHAT CAN YOU EXPECT TO LEARN FROM THIS BOOK?

1. In nature, when things are balanced, there is no disease! This book will help you find that natural healthy balance.
2. I will show you that observing, asking questions, and applying what you've learned are the benchmarks to increasing your knowledge.
3. Health goes beyond just eating a certain way. A healthy lifestyle goes deeper into who you are and how you are different from others.
4. You will discover the applications of yin-yang factors that will help you bring balance to your current situation and you'll learn how this knowledge affects your food choices.
5. I'll describe the paired organ system, and how the relation-

ships between the organs work. For example, we'll explore how the large intestine directly affects your lungs by using the five-element theory, which has been applied for over 4,000 years.

6. You will see why your body temperature plays a vital role in how you approach each meal.

7. I'll describe multiple factors that affect your health: biology, physiology, psychology, energy, and inspiration. Maintaining a healthy lifestyle goes beyond what you eat!

8. You will gain an understanding of the dos and don'ts to protect and help your immune system.

9. This book will provide you the awareness that you are your greatest investment! But you must be willing to participate in your own health in order to obtain this knowledge.

WHAT NOT TO EXPECT FROM THIS BOOK

1. If you are looking for ways to cure cancer, this book is not for you.

2. If you are looking for the holy grail or the magical pill that will allow you to keep your current lifestyle, this book is not for you.

WHO AM I?

I'm a podiatric physician and surgeon who is board certified in primary podiatric medicine with over twenty years in private practice. I have literally treated thousands of patients each year surgically, clinically, and naturally for toenail fungus, diabetes, gout, sport injuries, and various foot deformities. I can honestly say I have definitely seen my share of patients who have had diseases and illnesses that could have been easily prevented.

My career has taken me across the world to the Kingdom of

Tonga in the South Pacific, fulfilling a promise to my best friend in college that I would treat his people when I finished medical school. While helping those in Tonga on the medical mission, I saw firsthand the damaging effect of leprosy, elephantiasis, and club feet, conditions that you only read about in medical books.

Because I am always wanting to learn ways to help my patients, in my spare time I studied the art of manipulation through myopractics and energy application with Jin Shin Jyutsu to improve my clinical skills that have proven effective over the years. I love what I do professionally, and I may be the teacher with each page you turn, but I will always be the student at heart!

WHAT GOOD IS YOUR WEALTH IF YOU DON'T HAVE YOUR HEALTH?

We work our entire lives only to see our hard-earned money gobbled up by medical expenses. We might even experience a lower take-home pay from our current paycheck due to the cost of our monthly health insurance premiums. We are literally living our life reliant on remedies. Aside from the injury or traumas that may happen to us that are out of our control, we don't have to live life this way with diabetes, heart disease, and immune system problems along with other ailments we see later in life. I believe all of these things and more can be prevented if we'd only invest in ourselves and take preventative pathways. Yes, you are what you eat, and you will learn what I mean by this as you go through the book. You can use this book as a reference; you can even jump to the back of the book and just read the Immune Diet and start applying it, or you may want to reread it a few times from start to finish. There are no set rules here! Let's get started!

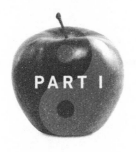

PART I

Primary Understanding of a Balanced Nature

CHAPTER 1

Do You Eat to Survive, Socialize, or Thrive?

———

Many people throughout the world are living the dream but paying the price for convenience. Does your present situation have any bearing on what you eat? I strongly feel it does, and what you eat today will indeed have an effect on your activity level and how you feel when you retire.

I have observed over my lifetime that "your health is your wealth." With that fundamental knowledge as a starting point, I have asked many questions. For instance, I began by learning what it means to say, "Chemistry is an assault on biology." Chemistry is anything that you put into your body that is processed or manmade that can be put in a box for consumption. Biology is every living cell in your body.

Obviously, health is a very important form of leverage. All too often, people do not appreciate the value of their health until they begin to lose it or until they are faced with a health crisis. As Robert T. Kiyosaki says in *Retire Young Retire Rich*, "How much enjoyment will retirement be if you are unhealthy?"

Here are some examples. The individual who just had a heart attack decides to quit smoking, or the individual who just learned they have diabetes decides to change his or her diet. Sound familiar? What I see most of the time is that there is a quick reaction, but then the remedy, "the pill," is much easier to swallow than applying a lifestyle change.

Every day, I see someone in my practice who makes these one of my statements:

- "I wish I could have…"
- "If I only did things differently back when I was younger."
- "I just found out I have cancer—so much for these golden years."
- "Ever since I retired, I have been in the hospital more than ever."
- "I am now on oxygen."
- "I thought once I retired, I would enjoy life."
- "I go to dialysis three times a week, so I can't travel anymore like I wanted to."
- "I am so exhausted; all I do is care for my ailing spouse."
- "We were supposed to enjoy our retirement years!"

I don't want this to be you.

One of the hardest things I deal with in a clinical setting is seeing patients dependent on medications to treat their present illnesses. It is not uncommon to see patients taking fifteen, twenty, or even twenty-five different medications a day to help control their diabetes, heart disease, and other ailments. All of these conditions and more could have been so easily prevented, in my opinion, if they would have just paid attention to the signs when they were in their twenties and thirties. But if you're in your forties, fifties, and even in your seventies, you can still make some amazing changes that will impact your health. Even though a majority of my patients are over forty, they still can benefit from changing their current lifestyle, but it is a lot easier to do when you are younger.

What good is your wealth if it all goes to your health? The system as we know it is set up to take your hard-earned money. When you retire, the system keeps you further enslaved into your retirement years. Think about it. You work to provide food for your family and to have enough money to pay your bills. Most people work to have some form of health insurance!

I'd like to help you understand a simple and easy way that will ease the fears of what your parents are going through or have gone through. It is a process and will provide a pathway to enjoyment in your retirement years. I cannot stop accidents, unexplained traumas, or injuries from happening. But what I can give you is the pathway to your peace of mind, knowing that living a healthy lifestyle is both beneficial and rewarding.

Healthy living has become a way of life for me. I am so thankful for a Sick Dad who allowed me to observe and ask questions. I am also very thankful to a Healthy Dad who allowed me to observe, ask questions, *and* who kept me on course as I applied the knowledge in my daily routines. Once I learned the proper way to eat, there was no more "dieting." Healthy eating became a way of life through a "live-it lifestyle."

INTRODUCTION TO SICK DAD

My biological father (whom I will hereafter refer to as my Sick Dad) was a robust, strong man for most of his adult years. After returning home from the Korean War, he took over the operation of the family farm; he knew how to farm, rotate crops, raise grass-fed cows, and never took a day off work. He worked the family farm providing for his wife and eight children. He spoke very few words and to have a conversation with him was all but impossible. In fact, the first time we actually had a conversation that lasted longer than three minutes was when I was eighteen years old and ready to leave home. I spent most of my time observing him when I was with him, but I was always eager to get in a question here and there.

He slowly aged, suffering with the pains of his heart disease, gout, and swollen legs. Sick Dad waited for his crisis to change, but it was too late. As I reflect on my Sick Dad, I often ask myself if I could have done more for him. Why didn't he listen to the principles I shared with him and why was he not willing to apply them to himself? The answer is simple: he asked me only a few questions regarding his health. I have learned that someone who does not ask questions does not participate in the process. This was my Sick Dad's situation. I wanted so much to tell him what I had learned, but when I did, it seemed like only useless words came out of my mouth.

WHAT DID I OBSERVE FROM MY SICK DAD?

Quite often while driving to the farm to feed the cows, irrigate the land, bail the hay, or to plow the fields, I would kick the empty soda pop bottles and candy bar wrappers off the passenger side of the truck onto the floor. On occasion, I would find his favorite cookies still in the cookie box, and I would eagerly eat one as it would break the silence while we drove to the farm.

Due to the lack of communication, if I was going to learn anything from my Sick Dad, I had to observe and figure out the answers in my mind. When I was lucky, he would answer one of my questions. Aside from being a good neighbor and a man who was very well-respected in the community, he loved his candy, soda, and ice cream. At home, we ate what my mother prepared, and usually, it was food that was grown from the garden and farm. At breakfast, I observed him pouring a large scoop of white sugar on top of his cornflakes. We commonly ate that cereal because it was the cheapest box cereal at the grocery store. I told myself that if my Sick Dad could do that, then I could, too. So I'd douse my cornflakes with several scoops of sugar. The highlight of the year came on Christmas morning when we were treated to a box of sweetened cereal.

When we would sit down at the dinner table, my Sick Dad would sit at the head of the table, then the eight children and my mother would find their places around the table. We did not have any fancy drinks. We drank tap water. We would have homemade bread rolls and some form of meat: beef, chicken, or pork. The vegetables were seasonal and usually came from the garden. In the winter months, we would eat canned fruits and frozen vegetables. The main vegetable was usually potatoes with lots of table salt and margarine. For dessert, we would have a bowl of fruit from the orchard. There was very little talking at the dinner table, as eating was just a stopping point for fuel to give us the needed energy to go back out and work. We were eating to survive!

If there was any excitement at the dinner table, it was when I would ask for a bread roll. As I would ask one of my brothers or sisters to please pass the bread roll, I would have to pay close attention as one would be thrown from the opposite end of the table. "Pass the bread roll" took on a whole new meaning!

After dinner, we would go back outside and work until dark. In Sick Dad's terms, "daylight is work time." Once it was too dark to work, we would go back home, and my Sick Dad would have his bowl of ice cream before retiring to bed. I rarely ate ice cream as it aggravated my asthma.

When I really started to see my Sick Dad's health decline was when he had his first heart attack in his mid-seventies. It slowed him down, but he still got up each day to go to the farm. Then the second heart attack came, followed by a third one. Finally, the fourth heart attack came, and then he took up residence in his recliner. I would make frequent trips up to see him, and I would recommend better eating habits, but he was set in his ways. The last time I offered any health advice was the last time I told him to lay off the ice cream at night as this was causing most of his gout attacks. He told me in no uncertain terms, "I will eat what I want to eat." I never again discussed my Sick Dad's poor health with him.

As I observed his behaviors, I asked myself questions. The main one was, "How did this strong man go from being so healthy to now having to use a walker to help him walk and being dependent on oxygen 24/7 to help him breathe?" If I had asked my Sick Dad if he planned on retiring this way, he would have laughed at me. Maybe my Sick Dad never planned on retiring, but I am certain that his dependency on oxygen and use of a walker didn't occur to him when he was still working in his twenties, thirties, forties, and fifties. On May 22, 2020, my Sick Dad succumbed to the illnesses that he developed during his very short retirement and left this mortal life.

WHAT I LEARNED DURING THE TRANSITION PERIOD

I want to tell you about the transition period from observing my Sick Dad to the time when I was introduced to my Healthy Dad.

As a child, I would see my Sick Dad's example and follow him. I would gravitate to the sweets and soda, but with my childhood illness of asthma and allergies that started around the age of four, I was limited in what I could do physically. Running and playing sports with the other kids in the neighborhood came with its challenges. Most mornings when I got up, I was so exhausted from the sleepless nights of just fighting to breathe. The only way I can describe it would be to imagine placing a straw in your mouth while inhaling and exhaling through it without the help of your nose and then doing this for hours.

I came to recognize that my asthma was exercise-induced, seasonal, and was usually escalated when I ate certain foods. As long as I had my inhaler, I used sports to combat my illness. At a very young age, I would ride my bike to the next town. I would record how long it took to get an asthma attack, and I would record what foods I ate that day. I was on a quest to find a cure for my asthma. Even though I didn't drink soda pop as frequently as my Sick Dad did, I continued to enjoy the sweets. It wasn't until I met my Healthy Dad and I saw what he did for my little girl that led me to asking questions about my asthma. The more questions I asked, the more ways I found to control and eliminate my asthma.

Patients often ask me why I chose podiatry over other medical professions. My response is that I broke my ankle in the eighth grade and the doctor told me I had a bone chip in my ankle. When I asked him if the bone chip could be removed, he told me not to worry about it. That left me with a void in my mind, wondering what effect that would have on my ankle in the future. What cautions should I take or not take? Questions like those drew me into my specialty.

YOU ARE WHAT YOU EAT

In elementary school, the bell would ring, and we would all line up in the cafeteria waiting to be served a hot meal for lunch. Each day, I observed a sign posted above the start of the lunch line: "You are what you eat." One day, thinking I could get out of eating my peas when they served cooked peas, I told the lunch lady that I did not like to eat cooked peas, only fresh peas. The next day, they were serving peas again. I said no thank you, but the lunch lady pulled out an isolated bowl of uncooked peas and handed it to me. I had no excuse now. I had to eat the peas. Trying to outsmart the lunch lady was beyond my creative skills. I accepted the peas and did my best to swallow them.

OTHER EXPERIENCES FROM MY YOUTH

I was once offered a cigarette by a man whose yard I had just mowed. After I finished mowing his lawn, I went up to the porch to receive my paycheck, and he said, "Son, would you like a cigarette?" Observing his very wrinkly facial skin and listening to his raspy voice and his deep cough, I declined his offer. I am sure this man had good intentions, but my impression at that young age of seeing his health was that his condition was something that I did not want.

On another occasion, I would sit on the porch with a good old friend, Mr. Maycock. I liked to go down to his place of residence. He would pay me a quarter per bucket of apples that I would pick from his apple orchard. But the bonus was, after I was done with my work, I would sit on the bench in his yard and listen to his stories about the good old times going fishing. We would drink Kool-Aid that was made with one cup of sugar and a packet of my choice of natural flavorings—"grape, raspberry, or strawberry"—and all we had to do was add one gallon of water from the faucet. It was so simple to make and tasted so good. Looking back on the summer on the bench, I realize drinking Kool-Aid was not the best thing for my health. But all I knew was that, aside from my asthma, I was healthy and active. The one thing that the Kool-Aid was doing to my body was the frequent visit to the dentist for all those cavities. The only other time I would drink Kool-Aid was maybe in college a few times when I wanted to add flavoring to my water.

Being raised in a small town had its good and bad. The good was, there was no fast food in my small town; the bad was, every time we had a school event that took me out of my hometown, I got to experience fast foods. This subtle habit of eating out at these places that I enjoyed came with consequences during medical school, as you will soon read about.

IN COLLEGE, I ATE TO SURVIVE

Looking back at my college years, I ate to survive, and I wasn't even aware of it. As long as I ate something, I was good. I would skip breakfast since sleep was so important to me. In college, time was more limited due to the demands of my studies. I had already mastered the art of peanut butter and jelly sandwiches, so that took care of lunch. Since money was scarce, for dinner, I became a professional chef when it came to cooking from a box of macaroni and cheese. Within fifteen minutes, I had cooked, ate my dinner, and was out the door studying again.

During the summers, I stayed active by planting more than 18,000 trees in Idaho and Montana for two seasons with the Forest Service. I also took on seasonal firefighting with the Bureau of Land Management for five seasons. Working at both places, my main meal for the day consisted of a Hostess fruit pie, occasionally a banana or an orange, and a sweetened juice or soda. On a few occasions, I would prepare something from home and bring it with me to work. If I was lucky, I would get a fresh doughnut for breakfast in the morning. Looking back, knowing what I know now, I would have done things very differently during my college years. I would have better selected my food choices. I would have tried to eat to thrive while trying to survive.

MEDICAL SCHOOL WAS THE TRUE TEST OF SURVIVAL

College was a cakewalk compared to the demands of medical school. There was no time for even the preparation of a fifteen-minute macaroni and cheese dinner. Those one-dollar tacos from Taco Bell at lunch along with Costco muffins and a root beer float were less time-consuming. My health issues did not happen overnight but came on gradually. The first year I survived, but in my second year of medical school, everything I was eating began to catch up with me.

THE WORST PAIN I EXPERIENCED IN LIFE

Being awakened in the middle of the night with a pain in my mid-back was the worst pain I have ever felt in my life. I went to the bathroom and was peeing blood. You can only imagine the thoughts that went through my mind: Am I dying? Do I have cancer? My roommate drove me to the emergency room. That's when the doctors confirmed I had given birth to a small but extremely painful kidney stone. The doctor gave me painkillers and told me that if there were other stones that were blocked, then I would have to have them surgically removed.

To make sure I did not have any more stones, I made an appointment with a kidney specialist. I underwent a contrast dye study to confirm my stones had passed. When I was told there were no stones present, that calmed my stresses and worries of the possibility that I may need surgery to remove the stones. Several months later when I had a week off for spring break, I used this time to attend my brother's wedding. I wasn't home for more than one day when I had another extreme pain in my back. My Sick Dad told me to go see the family doctor. I went to the clinic, and he recommended that I have a contrast dye study to see if the stone had passed. This turned into a major disaster, as I was now fighting for my life to survive physically as I had gone into a full-blown anaphylactic reaction just shortly after they injected me with the dye. By the grace of God and after extensive work by the medical team, I survived my near-death experience. I will share more about this in Chapter 12.

THE TRANSITION FROM EATING TO SURVIVE TO EATING TO SOCIALIZE

After completing medical school and my surgical residency, I ventured off into private practice. In the first few years, I was still in survival mode: skipping breakfast, eating fast food or having a pharmaceutical company provide lunch for my staff and myself. For dinner, once I got home, our family often went out to our favorite Mexican restaurant. I had no real concept of organic or real food. We usually purchased food in bulk and on sale. Over time, eating to socialize became more commonplace. My exercise was severely diminished due to feeling tired and exhausted all of the time. My body aches and pains were also more apparent. The kidney stones came back, and now I was also having lower back pain. I was facing a decision of whether to have back surgery or just push through the pain each day. What had happened to my body? Before, I was full of life, could fight fires, plant trees, and study for long hours. Now I was becoming more like my Sick Dad. I couldn't afford to take time off work because of my self-employment, but I knew I needed an alternative to avoid back surgery.

INTRODUCTION TO HEALTHY DAD

I'm always amazed when you project a thought into the universe asking for guidance and help and doors open up, which is exactly what happened in my case. I was told about a man who was trained in multiple disciplines of medical and alternative medicine who helped people with back pain without using any injections or surgery. His methods were based in alternative medicine, cranial sacral therapy, Jin Shin Jyutsu, oriental nutrition, manipulations, and attitudes and philosophies that produce good results for eliminating pain.

I made an appointment not knowing what I was getting myself into, and that's when my eighteen-year journey to living a lifestyle began. The first visit was very different for me, as I was so ingrained in modern medicine. I was always told, "There is a simple pill for everything, a remedy to take to make you better." I was so desperate for a solution because of the pain. I just wanted to have my freedom and life back.

After my first treatment, I had enough relief to continue my regular work schedule. I didn't visit the man again for over a year. He had given me a handout on nutrition that first visit, but to be completely honest, I didn't even look at it. "How could back pain be related to nutrition?" I would ask myself. I continued with the same lifestyle of not exercising and eating on the go "to survive" and eating out a lot "to socialize." It was about a year from the first time I was treated that I woke up one morning and could not even get out of bed. I felt so much pain in my lower back. That's when I called the man who had treated me in the past. He agreed to see me, and his treatment gave me the relief I needed once again.

You would think I would have learned that something had to change, but as I became heavier and my back became sorer and sorer, I resorted to more personal therapy of stretching and walking to keep me going.

As I would get my back worked on, my Healthy Dad would tell me, "Working on you is like working on a bag of potatoes. You are very stiff and dense." But somehow, he kept me going. This lasted for several years. As I would get worked on, he would throw out hints or comments on nutrition again. He would say, "Your body is so dense that it is so difficult to work on you. You really need to change what you're eating, or you're going to have a heart attack before you are in your forties." You would think a statement like that would change me, but it didn't until the crisis hit too close to home.

THE GAME CHANGER THAT CAUSED ME TO START EATING TO THRIVE

When my oldest daughter was around two and a half years old, she stopped eating. Having gone to medical school and with all my training in modern medicine, I was desperately searching for answers. Trying to find out why she was having so much pain when she ate, I took her to the emergency room, to the pediatrician, and had tests run on her, but still, nothing was helping her. This lasted for over a month. The feelings of being helpless and hopeless were beyond an emotional crisis; most of my energy and thoughts were about saving my daughter and not about myself.

I called the man whose work had already saved me from having back surgery to see if he could suggest anything for my daughter. He told me to bring her into his office and he would take a look at her. When I got to his office, I carried my daughter into the treatment room. I observed him using the art of physical manipulation which he was trained in. I heard a few pops in her mid-back. Then I heard the gurgle sounds in my daughter's tummy, and then my daughter sat up on her own.

She said, "Daddy, I'm hungry. Can I have something to eat?" Huh? What had I just witnessed? What did I just see with my own eyes? I was never taught this in medical school. I had worked with some outstanding surgeons and physicians and yet what I had just experienced was something that I had never seen before. I had been treated for my back pain with success, but I had just witnessed my little girl immediately healed after Western medicine could not provide me with the answers that I was desperately seeking. Taking my daughter into his kitchen area and giving her something to eat, still amazed at this experience, I turned to him and said, "Whatever you did for my daughter I need to learn. Can you teach me?" He said, "I will teach you whatever you want to learn."

My Healthy Dad, as I will now refer to him, started to first teach me nutrition and then eventually the art of physical manipulation, which is the subject for another book I hope to write in the future. He became my role model for living a healthy lifestyle. I had met someone who actually lived what they taught, and I wanted so much to learn what I'd just experienced. My Healthy Dad has become my mentor over the years in teaching me his profound knowledge. My Sick Dad will always be my biological father whom I continued to observe up until his passing.

My Healthy Dad's goal was to help me establish a good healthy body, so the first thing I learned was nutrition. He has always told me that nutrition is the foundation that one must start with to living healthy. Maybe that's why he was telling me in a subtle way I needed to change what I was eating when I first met him. I just kept asking questions and the answers kept following. It was several years before I was even permitted to work on anyone using this magical art of physical manipulation for healing. I learned more about nutrition, and I was applying it. I was doing everything I could to eat healthier. I had stopped all lunches with the pharmaceutical representatives at work, and I would no longer eat out at fast food restaurants. I brought my own lunch to work. I ate out for dinner less and less, and I was losing weight while building up my immune system. I was experiencing this healthy lifestyle and enjoyed newfound freedoms.

LEARNING FROM MY HEALTHY DAD

It was my focus to learn as much as I could from my Healthy Dad. So I invested the time over the next eighteen years to learn from my Healthy Dad. I would read the books he suggested and followed up by asking my many questions. I would take a week off each summer and go spend time with my Healthy Dad. We would have many discussions about nutrition and the art of physical manipulations.

For the first three years, I just listened and then applied the principles to my own life. I started to exercise more. I would buy more organic foods to eat at home, we ate out less, and I started to feel so much better. With each year in my training, I would be filled with more profound knowledge on nutrition. Slowly, over the course of the years, I was introduced to actually doing the art of physical manipulations that I experienced from being worked on myself and what I experienced with my daughter. This led me to continuing my studies of body manipulation and becoming a Jin Shin Jyutsu practitioner. I still work as a full-time podiatrist but greatly implement what I was taught into my practice. I have been able to see diabetics come off their medication and control their disease entirely through diet. I have treated fungal toenail infections naturally with success and adjusted ankles to take away leg pains. All of this training and knowledge did not happen overnight but has taken many years of studying and applying along with developing many of my own questions over the years. I still visit and have regular conversations with my Healthy Dad.

Presently, I can honestly say I have not had any back pain in years. I don't jump from diet to diet. Instead, I live a lifestyle that keeps me free from ailments. Today, I am pill-free. I can't even tell you when I last had an anti-inflammatory or a Tylenol. My waist size is back to the same size it was when I was in my twenties, and that's been true for the past fifteen years. I can perform my daily activities without pain as long as I don't do anything crazy or stupid. The fear of diseases really doesn't exist for me as long as I am actively living my lifestyle through good nutrition and movement. I have joy, peace, and comfort knowing the years ahead of me will be more pleasant from a health standpoint. I don't have to follow the same road that my Sick Dad took.

EATING TO THRIVE

Do we eat to survive, socialize, or to thrive? In times of crisis, it is my opinion we gravitate to the survival mode. We eat anything that will give us fuel to perform our daily duties. College was one of those survival times. When the COVID pandemic was announced in early 2020, I was informed there were massive lines of shoppers at Costco stocking up on food and groceries. I usually stay away from crowds, but I had to go to the local Costco and find out for myself.

This is what I observed (not to be confused with judging). I observed customers had their shopping carts filled with potato chips, sodas, alcohols, cereals, and all forms of meats from chicken to beef. Most of the organic items were well-stocked. Over the course of weeks, I noticed there were fewer organic items left to buy.

In good times, we eat to socialize. We go out for lunch or dinner and just enjoy one another's company without really paying attention to what we order or eat.

When I say we eat to thrive (which really means eating for our health), we are more aware of what we put in our body, and we spend a little more time finding the healthy foods that will give us the energy we need for our daily routines. Eating to thrive, you avoid the painful experiences of the medical ailments that creep up on us.

CONCLUSION

Most of my life, from my early days as a child to college, then medical school and into my surgical residency programs and even starting a family, I was eating to survive, with or without a crisis. I ate food as a fuel to get me from one day to the next.

There will be those who will say, "You're a doctor. How can you possibly understand my situation?" My response is, "I don't because we all come from a different storyline, but I know what it's like to eat cornflakes with powdered milk. I know what it's like to go to bed hungry. I know what it's like to sleep on a bus stop bench waiting for the bus to come first thing in the morning to take me to medical school."

I recall while in medical school, a homeless person came up to me while walking to medical school in San Francisco. He said to me, "Sir, could you spare a quarter?"

I replied, "I would love to give you a quarter, but I am trying to figure out how I am going to pay this $232,000 student loan bill." He then reached in his pocket and pulled out a dollar bill and said, "Here, let me help you." Yes, this actually happened, and although I never have been homeless, I can only imagine eating to survive in these situations is beyond what I have gone through.

This chapter was to get you to start to identify how you approach how you eat; do you eat to survive or thrive? In the next few chapters, I will show you how to protect your body's health while eating to survive. I hope I got your mind thinking. Where is your health today? Thriving or surviving?

I'm eager to get this information out to you, but first we have to start with the foundation of nutrition. I'm passing this information on to you so you can change what you are currently doing to ease the fear of diseases, labels, and ailments.

I'm all about prevention. It will be up to you, the reader, as to what questions you formulate and how you will apply the answers.

It is said that life experiences become our greatest teacher. Now, having gone through it myself and introducing it to countless patients over the years, I'm excited to share with you this way of how I was trained in nutrition. The focus of this book is on nutritional health. Therefore, the majority of the book will be the questions I asked my Healthy Dad, along with his responses. With the permission of my Healthy Dad, I am permitted to share with you what I was taught, what I learned, and how I applied it.

Are you ready to eat healthy to thrive? Or do you want to eat to survive? Or just to socialize? When you eat to thrive, you can also eat to socialize and survive!

Are you ready to dive deep into what really makes you go beyond the genetic markers? Why is it that you are different from other family members or even friends?

CHAPTER 2

Who You Are When It Comes to Your Health

———

What do the yin-yang factor, attitudes, the five elements, body types, and blood types have to do with you and your health? What makes you so different from others when it comes to your health?

In his spare time, my Sick Dad would put puzzles together to keep his mind active. I was amazed by how he would take a puzzle and put it together by looking at the box. What was even more amazing to me was how he did it upside down most of the time. In each of us contains the pieces to our puzzle. We are so unique and different to the point that it would be impossible to find another puzzle just like us. Sometimes we need to think outside the box to find the answers no matter how the box is presented to us, "upside down or right side up."

This chapter will show how we are different from others. We are indeed different from even our own brothers, sisters, mom, and dad. I believe that's why most diets work for only about six months before you have try a new one keep seeing results. By understanding who you are, you will have a better understanding of why things work and why other things don't. There will be less dieting and more living.

WHO IS THIS BODY WRAPPED IN SKIN?

To answer this question, we must lay a foundation as to why I am different from others. Why do certain foods agree with me when other foods do not? Why do some diets work for me but not my immediate family while other diets do not?

Here are five ways that will help you see why you are so different from others:

1. Yin-Yang Duality or Nature
2. Attitudes and Beliefs, "The Neighborhood Mind" (TNM)
3. Five Elements
4. Body Types
5. Blood Types

1. YIN-YANG DUALITY OR NATURE

The yin-yang principle is simple. When it combines with the five elements, it becomes a very informative and powerful tool for understanding ourselves. Once you are aware of this principle, you will want to live your life accordingly.

The two forces are always opposite and antagonistic. This is why in Chapter 3 I call it, "The Law of Opposition": "For if there is evil, there is good, and if there is sickness, there is health, and if there is hot, there is cold." This principle has been around since the beginning of time, and it's been in practice in the Orient for over 4,000 years. It is my purpose and intention to keep it simple and understandable.

Yin force is expansion, something that grows quickly and in great size but in a relatively short time. Yin makes us expand in ways physiologically and mentally. Elements that make us dizzy or lightheaded will be yin in nature. Things that make us cold, weak, and tired will also fall into the yin constitution. For example: water, sugar, alcohol, the fermentation process, raw, spicy, fear, and worry. Most people today have more of a yin constitution.

Yang force is contraction, stored energy life, and is heavy and dense. In the fermentation process, salt (which is very yang) will shrink the vegetables. If too little salt is used with the vegetables, they will spoil and eventually rot. The yang quality of the salt is what preserves them. The longer they are stored, the more yang they will become. Yang's characteristics are hot, full of energy, and active. Examples are salt, bitter, meat, dense, concentrated, and fire/cooking.

COMBINING THE YIN AND YANG IN WORKING TOGETHER

The activity of both yin and yang affects each of us in our innermost being. When you are cold, you want to get warm. When you are warm, you search for water to refresh yourself to cool down. This change from yin to yang can affect you adversely if you do not acclimatize yourself to the ever-changing conditions. That is why we should be careful to change our diet whenever we move from a cold place to a warm one and vice versa.

Whenever a person eats, it affects their condition to some degree. Just as the weather from the outside affects us, so does the food we eat, whether it be liquid, spicy, or acidic. This food inside of us can produce a sensation of being cold or hot; this is a key element in maintaining a healthy immune system.

A good cook knows one simple secret—yin cannot be delicious without a bit of help from yang. Salt, when added in correct measure, helps create the ideal taste. A potato without salt does not taste like a potato! The opposite is always needed to enhance one's quality. The wise person who has an understanding of natural attraction between yin and yang will not let their desires overshadow their wisdom.

When we are free to accept the two forces in the law of opposition, we are neither controlled nor overwhelmed. Rather, we are aware. The opposition is natural and the way nature intended it to be.

2. ATTITUDES AND BELIEFS
WHAT ARE THE ATTITUDES AND BELIEFS THAT AFFECT WHO YOU ARE, OR "THE NEIGHBORHOOD MIND" (TNM)?

We chose to come to planet Earth. We choose the day, time, and place, as well as the venue, or "The Neighborhood Mind" (hereinafter TNM). We signed the contract "True Purpose of Life," but when we went through the birth trauma, we forgot we signed it and forgot that we agreed to be here. That does not cancel the contract with our soul; it only makes it more challenging. So events in life are the fulcrums to catalyze you to seek to know the higher reason on why you are here and discover who you are to connect to your soul!

Pain is a motivator. This is the fulcrum of change. Sensations are the gift and blessing of this dimension. The important factor is that if you do not love yourself, because you have been told by others you're inadequate, you will react and not realize who you are. The attitudes come from outside of programming.

TNM is the subconscious program "teachings and beliefs" that are given to you by your environment. In other words, it's "the neighborhood" you grew up in and the programming given to you by your environment before you were old enough to filter it out! These are the people you are by, which go back seven generations, and the beliefs passed down to you from your immediate family and neighborhood.

By the time you are seven years old, 6/7 (approximately 85 percent; this is cosmic geometry) of your psychology or emotional nature has developed in this ratio: 25 percent in utero, 20 percent during your first year of life, and 15 percent the second year. By the time you have your second birthday, 60 percent of your psychological programming has developed, and in the next four years, the remaining 25 percent has developed! Have you heard of the "terrible twos"? This is when you start to reject outside input and try to create your own reality. So the word you use most as you start to reject outside input and instead attempt autonomy is no. But you are not old enough to go live on your own, so you learn to navigate the TNM by stuffing down your emotions and then acting out as you are not able to move out of TNM yet.

The environment of the neighborhood is comprised of the people, who can be divided into three main groups, whose beliefs and ways of interacting will dictate your programming. There are three primary groups in TNM: religion, government, and society. If 85 percent of your emotional nature/psychology is developed before you are seven years old, this is the programming you will react to for the rest of your life. You will develop all of your emotions and filter all of your thoughts through the beliefs that were given to you. This programming comes from seven generations back, to include 254 people: your parents, grandparents, great-grandparents, and so on.

WHAT IS THE OTHER ONE-SEVENTH OR 15 PERCENT?

The other 15 percent is what you get to decide after age seven. You will have the freedom of choice to either interact or to not react. At the age of seven, you are approaching the age of accountability. This is when you decide what you think and believe! You start to develop your own attitude about reality and to be responsible for your own beliefs.

HOW DO YOU CALCULATE THE NUMBERS?

You picked up all the emotional traits of your ancestors from seven generations back. What you choose to express, such as anger, grief, worry, fear, and trying, are the attitudes that create ailments and illnesses.

If you understood your parents' emotional traits, do you think you'd be a more harmonious person? Yes, because you would be more objective! Those traits are more of the emotional aspect within themselves. The traits express themselves in their physical ailments or attributes, which is not just genetics.

As I said, you pick up all the emotional traits from seven generations back. This means, if you act like them, you will have similar ailments or attributes. Maybe that would explain why Type 2 diabetes runs in the family or why some cancer and heart conditions run in the family. In Chapter 4, I will explain this in more detail.

Eighty-five percent of your psychology and emotional traits is from your ancestors' emotional programming. If you're angry, your (thought) DNA spirals back to one of those ancestors. If you're loving, you can trace it back to another (thought) DNA staircase.

WHAT ARE THE FACTORS THAT CAUSED THOSE ANCESTORS TO BE AFFECTED BY TNM?

Religion controls you by grief and fear.

Government controls you by anger and worry.

Society controls you by ego and desire.

3. THE FIVE ELEMENTS THEORY: AN OBJECTIVE ATTITUDE THRIVES AND A SUBJECTIVE ATTITUDE KILLS

There are six elements, but only five are used to treat or manage the primary functions of the body. The sixth element is on another level. It is the soul connection, or purpose of why you are here (also known as the dharma sutra or life's work).

- **Reaction**—"Subjective"—Five Elements of Attitude: worry, grief, anger, fear, and ego (sixth is desire).
- **Interaction**—"Objective"—Five Elements of Attitude: thoughtfulness, compassion, forgiveness, trust, and love/ acceptance (sixth is purpose).
- **Forgiveness**—Releases or takes care of the past: grief and anger.
- **Trust**—Releases or takes care of the future: worry and fear.
- **Thankfulness**—Releases or takes care of the present/pre-tense (pretending to be someone you are not: ego and desire).

THE DEPTHS OF DYSFUNCTION

1st Depth—**Worry** is sufficiency for the future—money, food, clothing, shelter, and warmth.

2nd Depth—**Grief** is communications in the past, which have not been worked out between people—comments and judgments.

3rd Depth—**Anger** is perpetrations in the past—physical harm and violence.

4th Depth—**Fear** is physical harm that might happen in the future—burn in hell.

5th Depth—**Ego** is trying to be someone you are not—king or somebody of high importance.

6th Depth—**Desire** is wanting something that you have not earned—money and fame.

THE FIVE ELEMENTS WITH THE ASSOCIATED ORGAN AND ATTITUDES THAT CAUSE DYSFUNCTION

1. **Earth.** Pancreas (spleen) and stomach are worry and thinking. They represent future tense sufficiency, which is tangible.
2. **Air/Metal.** Lung and large intestine are grief, doubt, and debate. They represent past tense judgment, which is intangible.
3. **Wood.** Liver and gallbladder are anger and frustration. They represent past tense violence, which is tangible.
4. **Water.** Kidney and urinary bladder are fear, anxiety, paranoia, and apprehension. They represent the future tense, which is intangible.
5. **Fire.** Heart and small intestine are ego and self. They represent pretense, which is intangible fire.

6. **Spark.** Pericardium and triple heater are desire and choice. They represent pretense identity, or titles/labels. All of this is illusion which is intangible.

4. BODY TYPES

Have you ever wondered why you are different from your other brothers and sisters or even your parents?

In the Ayurveda language, there are three body types: vada, pitta, and kapha. In the western hemisphere, people use the terms ectomorph, mesomorph, and endomorph. What does that mean? You are either thin, medium build, or heavy. There is no other way to say it. Stop and think: the last time you were in a group or crowd or in school and associated with other people, what did your eyes do? My assumption is, you looked at people and your brain formulated a judgment to the other person's body type. As human beings, we are so used to comparing ourselves to others. We do it with movie stars, we do it with models in the magazines, and we do it with fellow workers. The danger in doing this is we are now judging ourselves and formulating harsh thoughts that bring us down.

The three body types depict your mental and physical characteristics and your nature. If your characteristics become unbalanced, then we start to see disorders or diseases manifest. When this happens, your immunity depletes (lack of loving thyself), which opens the door to diseases.

The **vada** characteristic type is highly mentally focused. They are always thinking. They will have a thin, narrow body frame and are more sensitive to cold weather. They're quick to grasp information but quick to forget. They are more sensitive to pain, noise, and bright light.

The pitta type is more balanced. They will be medium build, athletically toned, medium strength, with stronger digestive characteristics.

The kapha type is more grounded. They are compact, strong, have a heavier build, have great physical strength and endurance, a desire for sleep, and are stubborn.

In the western hemisphere, there is a different language of terminology.

Ectomorph: Lean and long, with difficulty building muscle. Similar to the vada.

Mesomorph: Muscular and well-built, with a high metabolism and responsive muscle cells. Similar to the pitta.

Endomorph: Big, high body fat, often pear-shaped, with a high tendency to store body fat. This is similar to the kapha.

But did you know that most of us are not just one body type? We will fluctuate between one or the other, or we'll have two within us, and then some of us will even carry all three, but one will be more dominant. The point I am making is, you are not like your family even though your DNA (genetic makeup) tells you otherwise.

When you study these body types, you will see there is more to why you are different from someone else. If you want to study this topic further, I can recommend a good book that will give you a better understanding of body types: *Timeless Secrets of Health and Rejuvenation* by Andreas Moritz.

The main point is to accept your body type. Know that every

body type has both good and bad or negative and positive aspects. So embrace what you have.

5. BLOOD TYPES

There are four blood types—A, B, AB, and O. There are foods that are good and foods that are not good based on your blood type. I will keep it simple here. For more of an in-depth reading, a book you can read is *Eat Right 4 Your Type: Complete Blood Type Encyclopedia* by Dr. Peter J. D'Amado.

Have you ever wondered when you go out to eat with friends why one person will eat different foods than another? Is it because of the peer pressure of choosing a food item, or is it because there may be more than one blood type at the dinner table?

Type A do better with vegetarian foods and less proteins. They are the vada body types.

Type B do better with a variety of foods. They are the pitta body types.

Type AB do better with a variety of foods and more vegetarian foods. They are the vada and pitta body types.

Type O does better with denser protein foods. They are associated with the kapha body types.

To summarize, type O people do better with meats. Type A do better with grains. Type B do better with dairy. Type AB will be a combination of A and B. Your blood type is different from others, and this makes you different. It's one reason why a specific diet does not work for everyone.

CONCLUSION

This information is so much to think about, but to keep it simple, you are so unique that no one else can compare to you. Your pieces to the puzzle are so different and unique that nobody else has the same complete makeup as you do. Yes, you may have similarities, but there are still major differences. There are so many factors that play into what you ate or will eat: your blood type, your body type, your current state of emotion, your yin-yang constitution, your emotional ancestry traits going back seven generations, and the attitudes and beliefs within your own Neighborhood Mind. When you come to understand the interplay between all of these factors, you will realize how unique you really are.

Just because your father or grandfather was diabetic does not mean you will be diabetic.

Are you ready to accept who you are and move forward with a greater outlook on life and realize you are not your parents? The choice is yours. In the next chapter, you will read about why it is important to determine what to eat by just asking yourself, "Am I hot or am I cold?"

CHAPTER 3

The Law of Opposition

The Yin-Yang Duality of Nature's Approach

———

Is it possible to have a balanced life?

When I was beginning my studies with my Healthy Dad, he would always cause me to think of questions to ask. In this portion of the book, which covers yin-yang duality, I will shine more light on the matter and hopefully cause you to develop your own questions.

When I explain this concept that actually has been around for 4,000 years, I want you to think of what you were told about food preparation in respect to healthy eating and then see if there is anything different.

Healthy Dad said, "The yin and yang are an approach to making healthy and balanced meal choices."

The yin-yang approach was very confusing to me at first. Sometimes it appears to be so complex, which is why most people just shy away from it. But it is highly important and needed.

The yin-yang duality can be represented on a numerical scale. Here are some key things on that scale that we'll discuss in this chapter:

On the one side, you have the yin (weak) minus one to minus ten, and on the other side of the scale, you have yang (strong) plus one to plus ten. The closer you can get to zero is where the optimal health is located. If you notice, zero (balanced and neutral) is mother's milk (literally breast milk). I always wanted to have a T-shirt made that said, *Product of a breastfed baby! Purely organic at birth!* So what happened?

No matter how much we try, we will never be in perfect balance at the exact center of the yin-yang scale. However, we can use the principles of yin-yang to strive to reach that goal. This system of opposites is a "relative perspective dialectics" (see the chart in the section titled "What Is the Relative Perspective of Dialectics of Yin-Yang?") where we are in relation to the yin-yang or hot-cold polarity at the present time. With the use of this system of opposites, we can determine where we are to direct the application of where we want to be.

For example, if you are too warm, then you add cool. Balance will be achieved if the temperature of the cold matches the warm. So you have used the yin to balance the yang in a temperature relationship. This application of the principle can be used in all differentials. If you're thirsty, add water; if you're hungry, add nutrition; if you're tired, add rest.

When you are not as well-balanced as you would like, if you are too hot and you just go inside to the air-conditioned room, you may not cool as fast as you like, but in time, you may. It is not right or wrong, but it is still within the yin-yang principle. When you are hot and add more yang, such as meats, you will have excess yang. This will cause you to get grumpy and be hotter, which defeats the purpose of becoming more comfortable. This is still the yin-yang principle, and it's very important to your comfort and health. This is an awareness tool to give you choices you can make to keep yourself in balance and happy.

WHAT DOES THE SCALE LOOK LIKE ON A YIN-YANG COMPARISON?

The main goal is to be balanced, neutral, or zero in the yin-yang theory. Moving up the scale or down the scale to the opposite of what you are is needed. The scale starts at zero with mother's milk, and from there, you progress to yin or yang.

Sixty percent of the world's population is too much on the yin side of things; 20 percent are in balance, and 20 percent are too yang. There are gradients of yin and yang; the more extreme you are, the more out of balance you are. Please note, –1 yin is closer to the yang side of the scale, and the further out from zero you go, the more minus yin or plus yang it becomes.

When you are of the yin nature, you will be cold, weak, tired, and withdrawn. When you are of the yang nature, you will be hotter, stronger, more active, and more outgoing. In a health application, we will want to be in the mean average of +4 to –4 as these are the healthier parameters. The further out on the extremes you get, the harder it is to find the balance in the differentials. You will find most ailments are above +5/–5, or outside the +4 (yang) to –4 (yin) health range. By the time you get to 6 or 7, you will be taking medication or labeled with a chronic disease. Know that +10/−10 is so extreme that you will not be alive.

YIN SIDE OF THE SCALE AS IT RELATES TO THE THINGS WE CONSUME

−1 Yin	Rooted vegetables
−2 Yin	Stock vegetables
−3 Yin	Raw and fermented vegetables
−4 Yin	Berries
−5 Yin	Nonsweet fruits and lower-sweet fruits: kiwis, apples, stone fruits, bananas
−6 Yin	Sweet fruits: pineapples, oranges, dates, raisins
−7 Yin	Fruit juices, sugar
−8 Yin	Water
−9 Yin	Alcohol
−10 Yin	Chemicals

YANG SIDE OF THE SCALE AS IT RELATES TO THINGS WE CONSUME

+1 Yang	Beans, nuts and seeds, cow's milk, yogurt
+2 Yang	Grains
+3 Yang	Fish
+4 Yang	Eggs and cheese
+5 Yang	Chicken and fowl
+6 Yang	Pork
+7 Yang	Beef, red meat, wild game
+8 Yang	Dried types of meat such as jerky
+9 Yang	Miso
+10 Yang	Salt

Healthy Dad would tell me that cooked rooted vegetables are more yangizing than raw vegetables because we've added heat, so it makes them closer to zero. The further you get from zero or balance on the yin scale, the more yin or weaker you become. This is why someone who eats just strictly vegan will eventually run out of energy and will take longer to recover from simple things such as a common cold. How long that takes will depend on how yang you are before you become a vegan. A very yang person can do well to have a yin diet for a few years or, at most, a decade, before the yin will deplete the yang energy in the person.

WHAT IS THE RELATIVE PERSPECTIVE OF DIALECTICS OF YIN-YANG?

In this chart below, you will see many categories showing pairs of opposites associated with yin-yang duality.

DESCRIPTION	YIN	YANG
Gender	Female	Male
Tendency	Expansion	Contraction
Position	Outward	Inward
Structure	Space	Time
Direction	Ascent—up	Descent—down
Color	Purple–Blue	Red–Orange
Temperature	Cold	Hot
Weight	Light	Heavy
Factor	Water	Fire
Planet	Moon	Sun
Activity	Slow	Fast
Nature	Passive	Aggressive
Organ	Zang	Fu
Atonomic	Electron	Proton
Element	K, O, P, C	H, As, Li, Na, Mg
Biological	Vegetable	Animal
Agricultural	Fruit salad	Cereal, Beans
Season	Winter	Summer
Taste	Sweet, Sour, Spicy	Salty, Bitter
Voice	Delicate	Loud
Light	Darkness	Bright
Vitamins	B, C	A, D, K, E
Location	Arctic—Polar	Tropical
Diet	Vegetarian	Carnivore
Attitude	Negative	Positive
Expression	Peaceful	Anger
Pulse	Weak, Slow, Thin, Empty	Fast, Strong, Big, Full
Quality	Deficient	Excess

WHAT CAN YOU TELL ME ABOUT TRUE AND PURE YIN AND YANG?

True Yang	Wood, Liver—*Energy*, Strength and Movement
Pure Yang	Fire, Heart—*Heat* and Circulation
True Yin	Earth, Pancreas—*Sustenance*; Food, Shelter, Clothing, and Money
Pure Yin	Water, Kidney—*Water* and Cold
Balancer	Air/Metal, Lung: Can be yin or yang depending on the energy needed

This is to help you understand that there is a duality of the two types of yin and the two types of yang. The ability to understand the difference between the two will help you perceive duality within the duality. Keep an open mind as things will be explained through the material. It is important to understand more fully in this chapter and how it will tie into the next chapter on the five elements.

All of the components of yin-yang balance are connected one another, which is why this information is so important. A deficiency or excess in one area will throw the whole system out of balance. For example: If you want to put out a fire, you pour water on it. The pure yin helps balance the pure yang. If you want energy and strength, then you must give it real fuel, good food. True yin helps balance the true yang. If you eat really badly, then you are hurting the true yang energy. The true yin (nutrition) provides materials to store energy and strengthen true yang (liver). True yang provides pure yang (heart) energy to circulate the nutrition around the body, so the true yin (pancreas) ends up supporting the pure yang (fire). So if the earth does not have the nutrition or true yin, the consequences are that the liver does not have the quality of food to store energy.

Then the heart does not circulate quality blood, which will make you weaker, or more yin. A deficiency of true yin will create less strength in the body with regard to the wood–liver synergistic connection to the earth–pancreas (spleen). When you don't eat right, you will not have the storage energy, and you won't be able to sustain yourself. Nor will you have strength or true yang if you are not eating quality food.

When you try to do something without true yin, you use up your kidney chi (energy) or inherent chi to maintain the activity. That's because you're living on willpower and adrenaline, which uses up your chi. You don't have nutrition to accomplish the task (the activity you're involved in uses up all your true yin). It burns you out. You continue to function because you're running on kidney chi—pure yin, producing a heat symptom that is called febrile heat; defined as, when you're perspiring at a normal body temperature but have clammy hands and feet because of the excess fear/adrenaline causing perspiration. This is a sign that the kidney chi is low, and it is a pure yin "water" injury or depletion.

This depletion of pure yin is due to a true deficiency of true yin or lack of nutrition. You are using your willpower instead of living a good lifestyle. You are living on the kidney chi (the water element) by not putting in good fuel. Rhythm and pacing yourself are the balancers of the kidney and adrenal glands. On the yin side, these people will be weak, they worry too much, they think too much, they don't get grounded, they don't exercise, and the injury to the earth is lack of nutrition. This is what happens when you have a true yin deficiency and you still want to do things from the pure yin—"I will" by living on adrenaline. The cortisol or stress hormones are like drugs—sugars, coffee, chocolate, methamphetamines, cocaine, crack, and speed. These are false realities of energy! These are the extreme yin, which is so detrimental to the kidney chi needed to maintain life!

In this yin and yang, there are things that are good for you and there are extremes that are detrimental to the balance in the system of yin and yang. For example, if you just had a pure fire, you would burn yourself. If you have pure cold, you are going to freeze. The understanding of hot and cold is a great preceptor of yin and yang. Cold and hot and yin and yang respectively are almost synonymous.

WHAT IS DEHYDRATION IN RELATION TO PURE AND TRUE YIN AND PURE AND TRUE YANG?

Dehydration can be excess yang or deficiency of yin. An example is excess pure yang from external heat when you go outside in the summer without enough water. How do you balance excess pure yang? You add water—pure yin. But is the dehydration only a pure yin deficiency? Or did you just run out of sustenance and use up the pure yin causing internal heat—febrile heat? This is an example of true yin deficiency, electrolytes, and nutrition. Add it to get true yin into the cells to dispel heat from deficiency of true yin. There can be a deficiency of yin, not only just an excess of yang can cause a preponderance of heat; the lack causes a perception of more. Excess yang is not only when someone goes outside and they are hot; it can be a true yang—liver problem. If you have too much oil and fats or excess amounts of rich food, you're always warm, impatient, grumpy, or angry. This means your heart is pumping too hard, and you perspire with heavy food that increases liver congestion called excess true yang. In this example, the heart has to work too hard and that can cause an internal heat, which may cause a stroke.

THE LAW OF OPPOSITION

Reflecting on the material that was just presented to me, I posed a question to my Healthy Dad: "Is yin-yang like the law of opposition?" In life, we find ourselves looking for the perfect opportunities, the perfect companion, the perfect dress, the perfect job, but what is perfect? The law of opposition is just that when you have an opposing force on one end that is equal and opposite to the force on the other end. It is a force that wants to be neutral, but it will never happen because of the constant changes that occur in and around us.

It is a place called perfection (balance or in harmony), something we all strive for but come short in so many ways. We spend most of our time beating ourselves up because we are not there. Maybe this is why fad dieting is so popular. We all want to fit into that perfect pair of jeans or be a perfect weight. Then when we get into our older years, we just want to be healthy and not have to take so many medications. We want to do things and not have pain. We want to spend less time in the doctor's office. It is a cycle that is always moving and evolving. Having awareness of where we are currently today with our health today is a key factor. We can look into the future by looking at our parents. I am not saying look at their genetic component but at their lifestyle and belief system. What did they eat and are they happy at this present time?

The same is true with eating. We are either too far to the yin or weak side of things, or we are too far to the yang or strong side of things. Both sides have their effects. The yin is weak and tired, which in my profession manifests as fungal toenails or fibromyalgia patients.

Yin goes from –1 to –10, and yang goes from +1 to +10. Always try to find neutral. The goal of the lifestyle is directly situated in a place of balance or zero, where there are no extremes. Having the opposite brings us back to a neutral place.

The golden question in life is rather simple. From the time you get up to the time you go to bed, you should be asking these questions: Am I hot, or am I cold? Am I weak and tired, or am I full of energy? These questions should determine what you eat.

HOW DOES MY HEALTHY DAD EAT?

Eat with the understanding of what your present nature is—yin or yang. This concept is a key component so you can understand what your nature is. We talked about factors that make you, but the key is understanding the surroundings of where you presently reside.

If you are cold or cool, then you will want to eat yang foods. Yang foods are meats, salts, making sure to cook and/or warm solid foods. I'll explain this in greater detail in the chapter on "Live-It Lifestyles."

WHAT IS THE IMPORTANCE OF EATING FOOD COLD OR WARM?

If you are hot and/or warm, you will need raw or cooling yin foods to balance out the extreme of yang. With that said and depending on where you live, you will want to make sure your food and fluids are healthy and did not come from a place that was contaminated with bacteria or chemicals. In China, there's a reason why they don't eat raw foods. It's because they use human waste as fertilizer, so there is a bacterial problem in China. You would think this is not a yin-yang base principle, but it is. Cooking (yang) kills bacteria (yin).

HOW DO WE KNOW WHAT TYPE OF FOOD TO EAT AT ANY GIVEN MOMENT?

As a general rule, when you are sick with a yin cold condition, you need to have cooked soups and stews. When you are more yin tired and weak, you will need easy-to-digest foods like grains and veggies prepared in soups and stews cooked with a meat broth. When you are more yang and warm, then you should eat salads, fresh food, and consume more fluids, such as raw fruits and vegetables. When you are balanced, neither hot nor cold and are feeling good, you can have a variety of raw fruits and veggies and cooked foods.

I asked my Healthy Dad this question: "Do you know what the most common disease known to man is?" He replied, "Iatrogenic?" Nope! "Heart disease?" Nope! "Diabetes?" Nope! "Cancer?" Nope!

"What is it?" he said. I replied, "Excusitis. We seem to always have an excuse for everything." The great gift of life is, you get to choose what foods you eat. Choosing to eat the right foods by listening to your body temperature is vital.

HOW DO WE APPROACH THIS WAY OF EATING?

Here is a simple and basic question to ask yourself each morning, noon, and night: How do I feel? Whether I am hot or cold and feel good or bad will determine which way I gravitate to what I choose to eat for breakfast, lunch, and dinner. For instance, if I have worked outside all day and it is the middle of the summer, that juicy steak is not going to sit well with me as it is too warming. I will gravitate more to a salad and add some wild salmon if I want more protein in my meal. But if I wake up cold and tired, I will eat something warm and nourishing like stew or a cooked bowl of organic oatmeal with blueberries and maybe a little grass-fed yogurt with coconut milk.

IS THERE A RIGHT AND A WRONG WAY TO EAT?

Lots of chewing and small portions are best as you will digest the food better so it will not be fermenting improperly in the intestines overnight. Also, we need less food than we usually eat when we chew more. This will make you feel as satisfied as you would eating larger quantities because chewing twenty minutes is the time it takes to satisfy yourself rather than eating larger quantities of food. Also, the more well-chewed the food, the better your body will be able to digest it.

WHAT DO YOU MEAN BY YINIZING AND YANGIZING DIETS?

Most diets never really work because they are either too yin or too yang. The food in the diet doesn't adapt to the person for that day. Rather, it is a set protocol that does not incorporate an individual's nature of yin and yang.

There are many diets out there that claim to be the diet of the century, the diet that will fix all things and promise that you will lose weight and make your life so blissfully happy. All you have to do is eat this or that or take this pill. What I find is that most diets are only good for a short period of time before some form of ailment takes place. Yinizing diets eliminate all animal proteins and require that you eat mostly veggies, fruits, and juices. The yangizing diets are based on meat proteins like the Keto diets, but they will overlook the important grains and beans because they are high in carbohydrates. Carbohydrates are so important for balancing your blood sugar and improving your immune system. So without carbohydrates, over time, you will start to crave sugars to get energy.

HOW DO YOU KNOW WHAT YIN AND YANG ARE WHEN IT COMES TO THE FOODS YOU ARE EATING?

- Most yin foods are vegetables and fruits (nightshades), beverages, and especially raw and cold foods.
- Medium yin foods are yogurt, nuts, seeds, beans, and in general, cool foods.
- Most yang foods are meats, salt, dense, baked, and cooked foods.
- Medium yang foods are grains, eggs, cheese, fish, seafood, spices, and warm foods.
- Quick-growing and leafy vegetables are more yin—romaine, red leaf, bib, arugula, spring mix, bok choy, kale, spinach, and chard.
- Yang takes a longer time to grow—root vegetables, such as carrots, onions, rutabaga, turnips, radishes, beets, and green beans.

HOW DO BODY TEMPERATURES PLAY INTO ALL OF THIS?

Healthy Dad asked me, "How are you feeling? Hot or cool?" If your temperature is low, then you are yin and you're going to need warmer food and more yang-type foods. If you're hot, you need to worry about how hot the fire within you is, so you want cooling foods. If you have a very hot fire and you put some green or wet wood on it, it will not burn up, but you can burn up poor quality fuel with a real hot fire. But you cannot burn up poor quality fuels with a smoldering fire. If you put a bunch of green leaves on that fire and it wasn't really hot, it will go out. If you have a smoldering fire with smoke, it's like phlegm in the body, which is a symptom of yin.

Foods that cannot be digested easily will cause you to have gas, bloating, sinus trouble, and headaches. Foods that are yin will cool the fire. Healthy Dad gave me an example. When the fire will be too hot, it wants a little cooling. That's why the firemen get out the water hose and pour the water on the fire—to try to put the fire out. But if the fire grows really fast, the firemen have to stand out there and pour the water on the fire for a longer period of time. But if it's a really large fire, then water may not even work, and that's when other sources will need to come in and help. The true yin doesn't fix true yang very fast, but eventually it does if you are persistent.

You want the fire to happen, but when you want to control it, just put a little bit of cooling on it; true or pure is the question to know how to control it. After hearing this example, I could easily relate as I had spent five years fighting wildland fires.

Here is a good example. In the hot summer temperatures of Arizona, when you are working outside and then you decide to eat meat, you will be grumpy because the double yang (the body's temperature and meat) don't make a yin. Yang is grumpy and aggressive, and yin is passive. The yang person who eats hot foods gets dehydrated. They're going to be grumpy, and more than likely they're not going to be nice to their family when they get home. They are going to have problems in different ways other than what they are experiencing within themselves.

If the yang person were to drink water and eat watermelon and have some fresh vegetables, they would be cool and fresh and feel good and strong. They'd be able to sleep and be more pleasant when they got home. They will get up rested; they will be functional and alert.

In Arizona during summer, you need to be more vegetarian if you are working outside in the heat. You need to have more fresh foods if you're not having tremendous phlegm or congestion.

WHAT HAPPENS IF YOU LIVE IN ARIZONA OR A HOT PLACE BUT WORK INDOORS?

The fluorescent and blue lights put out an energy that causes your melatonin to be changed, so there's an energetic result. What happens is, people who are so yin in a cold climate or environment due to the air-conditioning inside and who hardly ever go outside and embrace the heat of the day, their bodies become more yin or weaker. Even though they are living in a hot area, they are not living outside or getting exposed to the heat because they have an air-conditioned car, with an air-conditioned home and workplace, and they are eating cold foods, all of which are making them more yin or weaker.

WHAT ABOUT THE NORTHERN COUNTRIES SUCH AS CANADA?

In Arizona, most people will eventually go outside and experience natural heat, but for the countries that don't have the luxury of being able to go outside, they will get really sick if they eat cold foods and the yin-type foods. Yes! The place where you live and work has an effect on you.

Your external environment has an effect on your ecosystem that has an effect on your dietary choices. In a cold climate like

Alaska, you don't see too many vegetarians. They'd die from respiratory-elevated pneumonia. But you don't see a lot of big heavy meat eaters down in the tropics either because it's hot. If they ate hot foods, they would be grumpy and they would be violent. They would be having accidents and they would get heart disease. Yin is the common nature. If you're cold, you are going to eat warm foods, such as soups, stews, and meats that are warming. Beef is the warmest followed by chicken, lamb, and then eggs, cheeses, and fish.

WHAT IS THE BEST FOOD TO EAT WHEN YOU TRAVEL TO A COOLER CLIMATE?

The first thing I will eat is chicken soup with vegetables and brown rice. When I eat chicken soup, it brings my body temperature up and nourishes me, and the prebiotics in vegetables and brown rice grow good bacteria within called probiotics. This sets the immune system to keep me balanced.

WHAT IS THE KEY FACTOR TO A GOOD IMMUNE SYSTEM?

When you have a good body temperature, you have a good immune system. When you are warmer, you can grow the right bacteria. This is why your body temperature is best at 98.6°.

WHAT ABOUT FISH?

Fish is more toward the neutral on the yin-yang scale than cheese, eggs, or chicken, all of which are a little more yang than fish. Shellfish is more yang than fish. Whitefish is less yang than redfish. Salmon is more yang than most of the other fish.

WHY IS SALMON THE MOST YANG FISH?

Salmon has the highest amount of good omega-3 fats. So your fattiest fish are more yang. The less fat it has, the less yang it is. Why can whales go deep in the ocean where it's almost 35°–45°F? They are full of blubber. They have one to two feet of blubber on the inside of their body. That's their insulation on their body wall.

CAN YOU TELL ME WHAT HAPPENS TO FOOD WHEN IT IS COOKED VERSUS EATEN RAW?

Cooked vegetables are more yang. This is why someone who is yin, tired, or weak will benefit from cooked root vegetables. In the case of a yin diabetic, the raw vegetables are too yin. This is why yang diabetics will benefit from raw vegetables as long as they do not have any respiratory conditions.

WHAT ABOUT FRUITS?

Fruits are more yin than vegetables. Whole raw fruit is extremely yin. If you're in Alaska and you're eating fresh fruits in the winter when it is thirty below zero, you're going to have lung trouble. Why? Because your body temperature, especially in your intestinal tract, is going to be too low, which is too cool (yin) to grow beneficial bacteria. This will cause you to get phlegm, and you will develop a respiratory problem that will turn into pneumonia. Do you see the connection? Two yins do not make a yang!

WHAT DOES IT MEAN TO HAVE A PAIRED ORGAN SYSTEM IN MEDICINE?

Paired organs are a synergistic system of essence and function, which equals building up and breaking down, ascending and descending, which are primary insights of yin and yang. The yin organ creates the essence, and the yang organ stores and uses that essence. This is the way the two organs connect in the elemental nature. In medicine, one needs to understand this to achieve health in the body. Once you understand the paired organs are connected, it is easily perceived how, for example, the lungs and the large intestine affect each other. They maintain your body temperature, which is why the lungs will not have phlegm. You eat to maintain the temperature of your body. The type of fuel you eat helps create your correct temperature, and then you can grow the beneficial bacteria and not get pneumonia. More discussion on this subject will be talked about in Chapter 4 , which covers the five elements and will show you how yin-yang ties into the five elements.

People do not understand the principle of duality that the concept of yin and yang gives them. Therefore, they do not realize the connection and importance of maintaining their health. Here are some examples of the pairs of the conceptual yin and yang duality of opposing forces that help you to maintain balance and health, but they are not limited to only these: hot and cold; inside and outside; ascending and descending; essence and function. These all correspond with paired organs. This is a true gift of understanding that is more valuable than money or possessions: "Health is your wealth." If you do not have health, you will lose your wealth.

DISCUSSION ON HOW WE STAY NEUTRAL

I was a healthy baby. My mother told me they kept me in the hospital a few more days because everyone at home was sick. It wasn't until my first vaccination at the age of four when I started to develop my childhood illnesses, such as allergies and asthma.

As I previously noted, mother's milk is where it all starts. It is the most neutral of all foods and liquids. It has proteins, glucose, and minerals. If a person is a 6 or 7 on the yin side of the scale and a vegetarian, they will need some yang to balance them; chicken or meat will be helpful. Someone who is too far to the yin side will need some warming products. Someone who is living on fruits and veggies will need some form of yangizing energy such as meats and cooked food. But if you're eating only meats, you're going to need some more yin—raw fruits and vegetables. Potatoes are more yin than other starches, and there is a lot of potassium in potatoes, so they are very yin.

Why do we put salt on our potatoes naturally? Because salt is yang. You see? We do things without even knowing why we do things. When we get sick and have phlegm, we think we are going to get better by eating a salad, but the reality of this will cause us to be more out of balance and we'll get sicker instead. When you understand what your body is telling you, you act accordingly. Yin and yang are the keys to knowing what to do.

CONCLUSION

Eating a balance of yin and yang throughout life is a basis for lifelong health. It's called a live-it lifestyle! The lifestyle is the true key to happiness and well-being, as "you cannot remedy a lifestyle." You must live it and not expect the extreme remedies like drugs, chemicals, vitamins, medical procedures, or even herbs and some natural remedies to keep you balanced. It is so difficult to cure an out-of-balance lifestyle, but it is easy to adjust a simple natural lifestyle back into balance, especially when you know the yin-yang and five element principles.

The main questions you should ask yourself each and every day are, "Am I hot, or am I cold? Am I weak and tired, or am I strong and full of energy?" This is how I start my day, and with each meal, I eat to determine what I need for that day. This is the main downside to diets. They tell you what to eat, but they never take into account how you feel that day. This has been my approach ever since I asked my Healthy Dad questions. Start asking yourself these simple questions and you'll begin to see the changes within yourself. This will be a key principle in retiring healthy! Where are you on the yin-yang scale?

CHAPTER 4

The Five Elements

If You Take Life Too Seriously, It Will Kill You

———

What if I told you there are other ways to run a check and balance on your body's system? Why is it that the first gout attacks happen at night, while heart attacks happen in mid-afternoon? Is there any correlation to having a poor immune system and respiratory infections?

While going to school, I used association as a method to learn material. When I wanted to remember someone's name, I associated them with someone I knew who had the same name. When I wanted to learn a lot of things for an upcoming test, I took those items and associated them with something familiar to me.

Association is a way to understand nutrition as far as our body organs and elements that are tied to those organs. Once you understand these connections, you will better understand how your body parts are associated with one another. For example, what does the large intestine tell us about our lungs?

There are elements in nature that affect us. These elements are energies; most people are familiar with the four elements (water, earth, fire, and air). The five elements have more dexterity and a variety of subsets of nature. When you observe these subsets of nature, you can figure things out.

There is an affinity: water has wetness, air has a lightness, fire has hotness, and earth has a heaviness. You can observe these elements of nature and learn how they apply to you in all circumstances.

For the purpose of this chapter, we will associate the elements with nutrition. The five elements are earth, air/metal, wood, water, and fire. In the western hemisphere, we associate air as metal. In those five elements, the only one you may not be familiar with is wood. Growing plants are flexible, and wood governs muscles and tendons. It is the one that westerners will have the most difficulty understanding.

When we are cold, we want warmth—fire. When we want air, we breathe deep. When we are hungry, we want to eat, and we use the earth element. If we want something flexible and strong, we use wood. If we are thirsty, we drink water.

By knowing that each element has a different effect on you, it's easy to apply these to change your health. Everything else will be a detail of those five elements. They will affect and have a consequence on your health. You can moderate your health by manipulating your body and by changing your diet or attitude system with these elements in mind.

ARE THESE FIVE ELEMENTS ASSOCIATED WITH ANY CERTAIN PLACE IN YOUR BODY?

The elements have energies or meridians, and they are associated with areas of the body. For example, if you look at an acupuncture meridian, you can see where the energy point falls on the organ meridian lines from where it starts to where it finishes. It is a reflection of both sides of the body: right and left side. When this happens, it correlates with thousands of functions that go on inside the body.

THE BODY MERIDIANS

Twelve Principal Meridians:

Stomach Meridian • Spleen Meridian • Small Intestine Meridian
Heart Meridian • Bladder Meridian • Pericardium Meridian
Triple Warmer Meridian • Gallbladder Meridian • Liver Meridian
Lung Meridian • Large Intestine Meridian

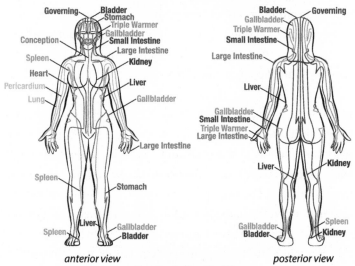

anterior view   *posterior view*

Two Centerline Meridians:

Conception Vessel • Governing Vessel

Meridians of the body: front and back views.

Then each element has a certain relationship with an organ; these organs are called the primary organs or the essence organs. You cannot live without these essence organs. They are essential for your body to function and for you to live. Earth is associated with the pancreas, fire with the heart, wood with the liver, water with the kidney, and air/metal with the lung.

When we think about it, the connections between the essence organs and the five elements are intuitive. Take the heart, for example, which is associated with fire. The heart pumps the warmth around the body, keeping the body at a certain temperature. It is like an air-conditioning unit in your house. If you want your body to maintain a certain temperature, you do it through your circulation, which comes from the heart.

Oxygen is an essence your lungs take in to provide your cells with energy, called prana chi. You take in oxygen from the outside and your lungs are the organ that allows you to inhale and exhale the air you breathe. This oxygen essence is from the outside and you compress it into the blood to combust glucose into another kind of energy, called nutrient chi.

In the water, you have the kidneys. The kidneys allows you to balance out the electrolytes and fluids of the body. So if you have a certain amount of minerals and a certain amount of water, you will retain that fluid by the way of the kidney, as it manages those solutions. For example, if you have too much potassium, you're going to the bathroom a lot more. Just like if you're too nervous, you will go to the bathroom more. It will be adaptive to the emotions as well as the physics. The kidney will balance the water in the body by maintaining minerals in the blood plasma.

The earth element is the pancreas. The pancreas creates an essence, called enzymes, that enables you to use your nutrition. One such enzyme is insulin. When you put enzymes into the digestive system, they will break down the foods so you can get the nutrition. When you put insulin into the blood, you can use the sugars, which are used for energy. The earth element governs nutrition and is also known as nutrition chi.

If you don't have one of these five essential organs, you don't live. Now, each of the five elements has a pair. If you look at the Five Elements Chart on the following pages you will see, for example, that the earth element is associated with the stomach and spleen. One will be called ascending (going up), and the other one will be called descending (going down). They dissolve and break down or eliminate things. The ascending ones are the essential ones for going up. They create an essence and build you up. You must have those to maintain life. Functioning organs are the managers or containers for the essential organs.

The heart is paired with the small intestines. The small intestine holds the nutrition and mixes the enzymes and the bacteria to be absorbed into the blood for the heart to circulate it.

The pancreas is paired with the stomach for an earth element. The stomach breaks the food down into a liquid. So the container of the stomach dissolves the foods and puts them into the small intestine.

The kidney is paired with the bladder, the container for the water. The bladder holds the fluids for a convenient time and holds the waste material from the kidney.

The lung is paired with the large intestines. The large intestine has the ability to absorb the fluids and digest your food. It also cultivates the bacteria to work on the food, which creates an ecosystem that is bacteria-rich and sustainable. If you maintain a good ecosystem in your intestinal tract, you have the ability to create good quality blood. It is the place where you maintain the balance to your immune system.

The liver is paired with the gallbladder. The gallbladder is the container of bile that is injected into the intestinal tract to break down and emulsify your oils so you can get them into your blood. The liver creates the digested bile where it is stored in the gallbladder. It works the same way as the pancreas and the bile duct, which aids in the breakdown of food so it can be dissolved and removed from your body.

All of the function or yang organs for holding, processing, or transforming essential nutrients into a form the body can assimilate. The pancreas creates enzymes to digest carbohydrates and proteins. The stomach contains the food to be liquified, as well as the enzymes needed to break down proteins and starches in the small intestine. The liver creates the bile to emulsify fats. The gallbladder is the container of the bile fluid, which is secreted into the small intestine to help with fat emulsification. When fats have been transformed into nutrition which can be absorbed into the blood through the small intestinal wall, the liver can chemically change the nutrients so the cells can use them.

The pancreas and the liver work in a similar way, as both secrete the enzymes or bile through the common duct into the duodenum which is the first part of the small intestine. These secretions aid in the breakdown of food so it can be transformed and enter your blood.

Below is a chart that describes the essence of organs and its association with its function organ. This is called the paired organ system.

PAIRED ORGAN CHART

ESSENCE ORGAN	FUNCTION ORGAN
Lung	Large intestine
Pancreas/Spleen	Stomach
Heart	Small intestine
Kidney	Bladder
Liver	Gallbladder

HOW DO THE FIVE ELEMENTS FIT INTO THE WESTERN MEDICINE MODEL?

Below, you will see a comprehensive chart that will tell you what each element governs in each category. For example, if you want to see the attitude of wood, you go down to the attitude listing and move across to the wood element, and you will see it is anger. Later in this chapter, I will discuss in greater detail what anger can do to your body. I did not go into details in regard to all the categories, as just this chart alone could take thousands of pages to be written on the subject and countless hours to discuss. This has been around for over 4,000 years and may ease your mind so all the information won't be so overwhelming as you'll be able to refer back to this table whenever you want.

FIVE ELEMENTS CHARACTERISTICS CHART

CATEGORIES	EARTH ELEMENT	METAL ELEMENT	WOOD ELEMENT	WATER ELEMENT	FIRE ELEMENT
Depth	1	2	3	4	5
Yin organ	Spleen	Lung	Liver	Kidney	Heart
Yin astrological sign	Cancer	Aries	Pisces	Scorpio	Leo
Yang organ	Stomach	Large intestine	Gallbladder	Bladder	Small intestine
Yang astrological sign	Gemini	Taurus	Aquarius	Libra	Virgo
Attitude	Worry	Grief	Anger	Fear	Pretense
Nature	Thinking	Logic	Emoting	Morality	Desire
Positive mood	Imagination Sympathy	Organizing Logical	Planning Decisions	Willpower Vitality	Joyfulness Activity
Negative mood	Indecisive Suspicious	Depression Judgmental	Impatient Aggressive	Insecurity Paranoid	Laughing Talkative
Color	Yellow	White	Green	Blue	Red
Age	1–15	16–30	31–45	46–60	61–75
Time–Yin organ	8:00 a.m.	4:00 a.m.	2:00 a.m.	6:00 p.m.	12:00 p.m.
Time–Yang organ	10:00 a.m.	6:00 a.m.	12:00 a.m.	4:00 p.m.	2:00 p.m.
Tissue	Muscle tendon	Skin	Blood	Bones	Blood vessels
Season	Late summer	Fall	Spring	Winter	Summer
Climate	Dampness	Dryness	Wind	Cold	Hot
Sound	Singing	Weeping	Sighing	Groaning	Laughing
Taste	Sweet	Pungent	Sour	Salty	Bitter
Odor	Fragrant	Rotten	Rancid	Putrid	Burned
Strain	Sitting	Lying	Eye strain	Standing	Walking

CATEGORIES	EARTH ELEMENT	METAL ELEMENT	WOOD ELEMENT	WATER ELEMENT	FIRE ELEMENT
Orifice	Mouth	Nose	Eye	Ear	Tongue
Bodily liquid	Saliva	Snivel	Tears	Urine	Sweat
Branches	Lips	Breath	Nails	Head hair	Body hair
Finger JSJ	Thumb	Ring	Middle	Index	Little
Treatment	Diet	Breath	Psychology	Physical	Inspirational
Physical change	Sobbing	Coughing	Gripping	Shivering	Anxious
Textures	Gummy	Rocky	Fluffy	Gurgles	Pulse
Direction	Center	West	East	North	South
Skin color	Yellowish	Whitish	Greenish	Grayish	Reddish
Density	Condensation	Solid	Gas	Liquid	Plasma
Energy	Downward	Solidified	Upward	Floating	Active
Note	G	E	C	F	A
Question	Who	What	Which	Where	When
Day of week	Saturday	Friday	Thursday	Wednesday	Tuesday
Moon phase	New moon	Waning	Waxing	New moon	Full moon
Planet	Saturn	Venus	Jupiter	Mercury	Mars
Food category	Carbo-hydrates	Proteins	Fats	Salts	Stimulants
Animal food	Beef	Poultry	Game	Pork	Lamb
Grains	Millet	Rice	Wheat	Beans	Corn
Vegetable	Round plants	Small plants	Sprouts	Roots	Large leafy
Fruit	Sweet	Apple, Pear	Stone fruits	Berries	Melons

All five elements act like a clock. On this clock, there are dials, and they all must work together. The minute hand and second hand all represent a balance of time that you can manage. In the case of the five elements, it is a management of your life. If the five elements are all working well, you are healthy. If one is not working well, you are not healthy.

HOW DOES THE PANCREAS INTERACT WITH THE STOMACH IN THE EARTH ELEMENT?

The pancreas secretes enzymes in the stomach/duodenum. The stomach holds the food until it is dissolved. This process of interaction works on digesting the foods; otherwise, enzymes cannot break down the food. The digestion begins in the mouth when you chew your food. If you don't chew your food well, the stomach will add hydrochloric acid (HCL) to complete the liquification. If you are too weak, or "yin," however, you will not have enough HCL to liquefy the food. You will have to be more particular about how you prepare your food and the types of food you eat. The older you get, the less your stomach can produce HCL (yang) and the less capable your body will be of digesting food.

HOW DOES THE LARGE INTESTINE INTERACT WITH THE LUNG IN THE AIR/METAL ELEMENT?

If you look at the lung as an oxygen-absorbing organ, when you have phlegm in the lung, it reduces that ability. One main thing to understand about the lung is it needs to be moist to absorb oxygen but not wet or damp. If you don't have phlegm in the lung, you can breathe better. Where does the phlegm come from? It is the imbalance of the bacteria and digestion in the large intestine. The large intestine also needs to be moist but not dry. You will want to connect the lung and large intestine to the proper balance of liquid in these two organs.

When you have poorly digested food in your large intestine, such as chemicals, pathogens, and junk food, it is difficult to break down the food and it will sour. The chemistry in the large intestine will be off, so the good bacteria won't be able to grow. The body's immune system kicks in and creates a white blood cell called a lymphocyte to go after the fungus, mold, virus, or bad bacteria. When mucus is formed to help eliminate the pathogens out of the body, it is called phlegm. This mucus will form on the internal surfaces of the lung and large intestine system of your body which causes you to have congestion in the lungs, in the sinuses, and even in the eustachian tubes. It is called pneumonia when the lungs fill up with phlegm and cannot exchange the oxygen.

I have seen a person who was told that he had congestive heart failure when he went to the hospital. But his ill health was due to difficulty in breathing because he lived off too many cold foods. His body got too cold and the good bacteria could not grow, which resulted in too much phlegm, which led to respiratory congestion, which led to heart stress. What happened? When we used the principles of yin and yang and the five elements to understand his condition, we realized it was a lack of oxygen, not heart failure. When we established balance in the digestive system, the fluid on the lung went away and his heart was okay.

Fowl is warming, which is good for the lungs. He ate chicken soup with no starch and no additional protein. It included some vegetables for roughage and some ginger for warming or heat. Within three days, he was out of the hospital, and in two weeks, he was strong enough to travel.

HOW DOES THE LIVER INTERACT WITH THE GALLBLADDER IN THE WOOD ELEMENT?

The gallbladder is a function organ that stores bile. When

your liver is congested because you have been eating too many low-density lipids (LDL) in junk food, which are high in hydrogenated fats that are undigestible to the liver, you will have a backup in the liver. Your liver has 20 percent of your total blood supply going through it every thirty seconds. So in order for the blood to get through the congestion, the heart will have to pump harder to force the blood through, which will raise your blood pressure. This congestion of the liver reduces the bile production, and now there will not be enough bile in the gallbladder to break down or emulsify the fats. Also, if you have a plugged-up gallbladder, which is usually from a gallstone or sludge, you will have less fat digestion.

HOW DOES THE KIDNEY INTERACT WITH THE BLADDER IN THE WATER ELEMENT?

The bladder is a reservoir for your kidney's waste products. It is the container for convenience, so it is a socially correct organ. In other words, you can go to the bathroom instead of your urine leaking out all of the time. It is an organ that makes you function better in your life.

HOW DOES THE HEART INTERACT WITH THE SMALL INTESTINE IN THE FIRE ELEMENT?

This is the most complicated for the westerner to understand because they do not associate the heart with digestion. The reason why the heart has so much trouble is due to bad foods. If you eat too much or have too much volume of stuff in your small intestinal tract, you are now going to have trouble with your heart. This is the main reason why they tell you not to go swimming after you eat.

The small intestine is twenty-four feet long and it has a lot of blood vessels in it. So right after you eat, you're sending about one-third of your blood to the stomach and into the digestive system, or in the small intestinal tract (which will get about 80 percent of that blood). This causes a pooling of blood in your small intestine, which causes a lack of blood in the muscles that you need in order to swim. The heart will have to produce more volume from a mechanical standpoint—that is, you will need a lot more blood to send enough to the muscles of the extremities and to the digestive system to process the food in your small intestine. When you're overweight, the body will need more oxygen, and the heart will have to pump more to keep the body oxygenated and nourished.

WHAT IS THE RELATIONSHIP OF THE FIVE ELEMENTS WITH THE ATTITUDE (WORRY, GRIEF, ANGER, FEAR, AND EGO)?

Physiophilosophy, or the knowledge that the thoughts affect the body, demonstrates that these elements affect every level of reality:

1. **Water / Physiology**—Which areas of the body and which organ meridian they govern.
2. **Earth / Biology**—What function they perform in health to keep your body alive.
3. **Wood / Psychology**—What attitude or reactive emotion a person expresses.
4. **Metal or air / Energy**—What electromagnetic energy has to do with your health.
5. **Fire / Inspiration**—What reasons you have to live.

The five elements are the key to managing imbalances in all areas of your life by recognizing the natures: wood, fire, air/metal, water, and earth.

WHAT IS THE EARTH (PANCREAS/STOMACH) EMOTIONAL ELEMENT?

The earth element is worry and thinking. They are the emotions associated with the pancreas/spleen. This is the concern about the sufficiency for the future: do you have enough food, money, clothing, shelter, and warmth? These are external applications to the body, which are tangible. Sugar is a placation for love, which will injure the earth element. The earth element is one of three chi you have. The nutrient chi is responsible for the integrity of the blood vessels and tissues. When you spend energy worrying about something you do not have, this will result in a loss of energy. You can burn up more calories worrying than you can by exercising because you elevate your adrenaline and use up the blood sugars stressing about things that may never occur. Consequently, you waste a lot of energy and deplete your earth element.

This is classic in diabetes, which is a consequence of using up too much insulin, and then you become too weak because you have given worry all the energy. What happens is, you will not have enough insulin to get the sugar out of the blood, which causes more acidity, and then your muscles will cramp. In extreme situations, this could cause a heart attack. Sugar is very abrasive to the vascular system. When elevated sugar levels are in the blood, it's like taking sandpaper to the blood vessels which creates inflammation. Bruising easily is the classic symptom of elevated blood sugar. In order to prevent this, you have to have enough insulin to reduce sugar in the blood, which diabetics don't have!

To recap, if you worry too much, think too much, or have a lack of self-love, this can cause you to worry more. When this happens, your body uses up the insulin by taking in sweets. Then when you use adrenaline for false energy, you increase your sugar metabolism. If you continue this, the pancreas will get tired and can't do the work to produce enough insulin. That's when you get sick, and it is called diabetes.

Sugar and sweets are a replacement for love. When you don't get the love you want, you find another way to get it with sweets. When you don't have unconditional love and just conditional love (attitudes), this leads you to attack yourself by eating poorly, which elevates insulin and injures the pancreas. If you don't love yourself, your immune system will literally attack the pancreas. This is a consequence of someone telling you that you are inadequate, that you're not good enough, that you're not fit enough, that you don't look right, that you aren't able to do this or that. These attacks occur when you don't receive approval from the person you're seeking the love from—The Neighborhood Mind (TNM)!

WHAT IS THE AIR/METAL (LUNG/LARGE INTESTINE) EMOTION?

The air/metal emotions are grief, doubt, and debate, which are past tense. Judgment is intangible or subjective.

Grief is rooted in communications in the past that have not been worked out with another individual. Grief, judgment, and doubt are the guilt programs where you debate yourself. This goes with the air/metal meridian, which is the intellect of the legal system. The law of lady justice is air, and air is communication because air is where you express yourself. In the air, if you have clear expression, you will have better health. The third thoracic vertebra associated with the nerve supply to the lung is one of the three energies or chi, also called the oxygen compression—"lung chi" or "prana chi." Grief will sour the mash (spoil or putrefy the chyme or liquefy the food) causing the bacteria not to proliferate, which will injure the immune system.

WHAT IS THE WOOD (LIVER/GALLBLADDER) EMOTIONAL ELEMENT?

The wood element is associated with anger, frustration, and impatience, which are past tense, and violence and physical harm, which are tangible. These are spontaneous reactions. These are directed martial or militant energy, aggressive and explosive. The liver is the storehouse of chi in the form of glucose, blood purifier, and as the organ that does fat metabolism and hormone balance. Congestion of the liver from eating bad fats will create a tension in the anger emotion, which will cause a person to react violently to circumstances. This is usually called a crime of irrational behavior. In extreme crimes, it is called second degree murder as it is spontaneous.

WHAT IS THE WATER (KIDNEY/URINARY BLADDER) EMOTIONAL ELEMENT?

The water element is linked to fear, anxiety, stress, and paranoia. Fear is a future tense, a physical harm that is going to happen in the future but has not yet happened. Fear is intangible. Fear elevates adrenaline. Trust is rhythm, routine, and pace. Fear is the opposite—apprehensions, uncertainties, and unknowns.

The kidney element is concerned for survival. The primary survival concern is the most basic instinct. Fear is the apprehension of something going to happen to you, which triggers the flight-or-fight mechanism. This is where you pump a lot of adrenaline which will cause you to use up all your sugar and deplete your insulin. Now you'll want to stay alive, but you don't have enough nutrient chi to maintain your ability to survive, so you will use your willpower in the form of adrenaline or kidney chi. Your kidney chi is your inherent chi—willpower; this is your inherited energy from your ancestors. It is the proverbial cup of energy given to you at birth.

You manage the three chi to maintain your daily activity. Did you take enough from the outside energy (nutrient and prana chi) today to not tap into the inherent chi? If you don't, you start to use the kidney chi up one drop at a time. Today, most people will have less than one-third of a cup of inheritance chi (innate vital energy from ancestors) by the time they are in their forties, so by the time they are in their sixties, they will not have enough energy to enjoy life and ambition to go out to play. This loss of chi will weaken this desire, which will be the onset of depression that suppresses the fire meridian, so their heart's desire will be diminished.

Most people had more energy when they were young because their cup was fuller. They used up too much energy by their thirties because they lived on sugar, stimulants, and adrenaline. This is hollow or false chi, which uses up the kidney chi. Now in their forties, they start to realize they have less energy. They are not present. They don't have willpower anymore, and desire is gone. I wonder how many drops of kidney chi I used in writing this book. Then when people approach their fifties and sixties, they will have heart problems. In their later years, they don't have enough vitality. This is a human tragedy! All of their energy was used up in their youth. People live on their willpower because they had a lifestyle of poor nutrition and a detrimental pace of life.

Healthy Dad went on further and said, "When one manages

the three chi with a proper lifestyle, then in your seventies you will still be able to do things that you want to do, providing you didn't have any major trauma, accidents, or injuries."

As long as you guard the kidney chi with good nutrition, quality of oxygen, and proper rest and exercise, you will have energy to enjoy retirement.

WHAT IS THE FIRE (HEART/SMALL INTESTINE) EMOTIONAL ELEMENT?

The fire element is hope, ambition, desire, and joy along with the ego and self. Fire is intrinsic, which is elusive; you can see the fire, you can feel the fire, but you cannot grab it. Earth, air, wood, and water can be put in a bottle and be contained, but you can't bottle or contain fire. With air, however, you can't see it; whereas with fire, you can. Try to put fire in a bottle and it is gone; it's the most elusive element. Fire is the internal passion for doing something. The fire element goes with premeditated activity or intentions. Intentions are the creator, and if you have a criminal intent to kill someone, it is considered first degree murder, which is a heart derangement.

Someone who has heart disease will have an imbalance in one or more of these meridians: gallbladder, small intestine, kidney, liver, the heart itself, or the will to live (purpose). These elements all work together like a clock mechanism. Hope is the critical factor of the heart that gives you the desire to continue to live. It comes from within you.

Hope is so important. Without it, you will be depressed and withdrawn from life. The remedy for depression is hope in the heart. It's not just chemistry, but there are some helpful elements of chemistry. Nutrients such as DHA and iodine create a higher metabolic rate in the brain, resulting in happy enzymes in the brain or endorphins that create that joy in life. In turn, these make you curious, which increases the activity of the hypothalamus, which then triggers the thyroid to increase its activity to speed up the metabolic rate.

Passion, hope, and joy will create more intracellularly metabolic activity. This all comes from your internal drive to want to do something. It comes from the desire to go play, so if you don't have the energy, willpower, or kidney chi, you won't want to do any activities. This is known as depression or the lack of hope. Random, joyful motion of dance is the best remedy for depression.

Hope says, "I can do this," so "I can"; depression says, "I do not want to do this" so "I don't." These attitudes will change your brain's chemistry. Attitudes are the key.

WHAT CONTROLS EACH ATTITUDE AND EMOTION AS IT RELATES TO TNM?

I referenced this in Chapter 2, but to show you the importance of attitude and emotion as it relates to TNM again (as a reminder, TNM makes up 85 percent of your thoughts):

Religion controls our grief and fear; beliefs are 70 percent of all your thoughts from TNM.

Government controls our anger and worry; laws are 10 percent of all your thoughts from TNM.

Society controls our ego and desire; approvals are the remaining 5 percent of your thoughts from TNM.

HOW DO YOU RELEASE THE ATTITUDE AND EMOTIONS?

Forgiveness releases or takes care of the past; grief and anger.

Trust releases or takes care of the future; worry and fear.

Thankfulness releases the pretense; ego and desire, sixth depth, pretending to be someone you are not, and wanting something that is not yours.

WHAT CAN YOU TELL ME ABOUT THE THREE ENERGIES?

There are three energies or chi in the body: **pancreas, lung**, and **kidney**.

1. The Grain Compression—Pancreas—Earth Element—Nutrition Chi
2. The Oxygen Compression—Lung—Air/Metal Element—Prana Chi
3. The Inheritance Chi—Kidney—Water Element—Willpower Chi

You have these three energies in your body. They are managed, balanced, and controlled by the function meridian, also known as the triple heater meridian. If you don't have enough of one, you will deplete one of the other energies: pace of life (kidney), good oxygen (lung), or good nutrition (pancreas). If you want to do something and have not fortified your daily intake from earth and air/metal, you will now have to go and take from the water. Once you get your portion of inheritance chi, you don't get any more, so guard your kidney chi.

One of the important goals in life is to protect that inheritance chi by not spending all of it before you get to retirement years.

If you maintain this energy chi when you're young, when you get older, you will have a nice retirement. If you don't, you won't. Plain and simple. The last breath you take is the last drop of the kidney chi in the cup you have left to spend. Save that cup, guard that cup so you can keep it full most of your life. Then as you get older, you will still have energy and a happy life. When you eat right and pace yourself, you protect that kidney chi.

The Western medicine and alternative folks think you can just go get some internal chi from elsewhere. This is a tragedy because you can only get the external energy, not the internal energy, so protect that chi!

WHAT IS THE TIMING OF THE ELEMENTS?

Each organ has a time of day when its activity is at a peak. It is a time where you restore the element/organ/meridian. For example, even though we breathe all day long, the lung has an active peak period from 3:00 a.m. to 5:00 a.m., peaking at 4:00 a.m. Please refer to the chart below.

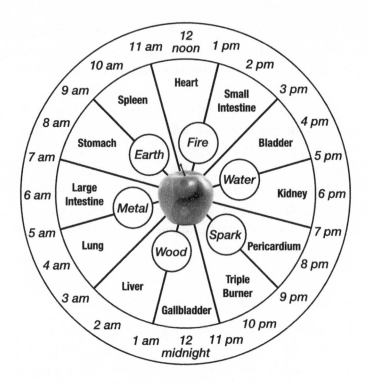

Here are timing examples:

- **Water.** If you are having a problem between 5:00 p.m. and 7:00 p.m., then you are having a weakness in the kidney energy.
- **Fire.** If you are having problems between 11:00 a.m. and 1:00 p.m. with a peak of 12:00 p.m. (noon), then you are having a weakness in the heart energy. If you get tired after you eat at 2:00 p.m., then you have a weakness in the small intestine meridian.
- **Wood.** If you wake up every night at 2:00 a.m., then you know you have liver trouble from 1:00 a.m. to 3:00 a.m. When you are angry at night, it will disturb the liver energy. It is best to eat at least four hours before going to bed so

the liver can clean and restore the energy without having to process extra foods or chemicals.

Most heart attacks happen in the afternoon. Of course, that does not mean a heart attack can't happen at other times, but in general, most heart attacks will happen between the hours of 12:00 p.m. and 4:00 p.m. (heart–small intestine association). My Sick Dad passed away at 4:40 p.m. due to heart failure. Most gallbladder attacks happen between the hours of 2:00 a.m. and 4:00 a.m.

THE ELEMENTAL STRESS ON THE NATURES

- Sitting places stress on the pancreas because motion is needed to mix the enzymes.
- Lying down places stress on the lung because you do not breathe deep and it lowers the oxygen.
- Eye strain places stress on the liver because the liver stores glucose and the eyes take a large volume of it to see. So you need to have a ready supply available.
- Standing places stress on the kidney because it stresses the low back and the knees.
- Walking/running places stress on the heart because it has to work harder.

Let's say you have a fever at 5:00 p.m. because you were working outside all day and you are now dehydrated. You add pure yin (water) and it goes away. But if you have a fever when you lie down at 4:00 a.m., you are having trouble in your large intestines, and then you need to have an enema to break the fever.

I began to reflect on my own experience from what I had learned from my Healthy Dad. I once had a patient who went into the hospital for extreme difficulty with breathing. The doctors were ready to sedate him and put him on a respirator in the ICU. I asked the primary care doctor, "When was the last time the patient had a bowel movement?" When they looked at the records, he had not had a bowel movement in days. I said, "Once he has regular bowel movements, his lungs will start working better." I received a call a few days later from the doctor, who informed me that once the patient had a bowel movement, he started to breathe on his own.

When I was in medical school and working on cadavers, the bodies that we were allowed to work on had a cause of death attached to them. I was amazed at how many people that had pulmonary arrest as the cause of death had a blockage in the large intestine. I was not aware of this knowledge back then, but somehow, I was able to correlate the two working together.

WHAT IS THE EFFECT OF THE RELATIONSHIP BETWEEN EACH ELEMENT AND ITS ORGAN?

There are two types of relationships where one organ supports another one. The first is the called the "mother-son relationship"; the **immediate** organ/element preceding supports the following one.

Examples of mother-to-son direct nourishing and strengthening relationship:

Fire (heart) strengthens earth (spleen), which strengthens metal (lung), which strengthens the water (kidney), which strengthens the wood (liver), which strengthens the fire (heart).

Grandfather-grandson indirect relationship: **two** organs/elements preceding support the **second** organ following one.

Example of the grandfather-to-grandson indirect awareness and supporting relationship:

The fire (heart) supports air/metal (lung), which supports wood (liver), which supports earth (spleen), which supports water (kidney), which supports fire (heart).

Now when you add the elements, attitudes, and emotional stresses into the picture, you will see how this simple chart will show you avenues to overcome an injured liver due to anger, an injured kidney due to fear, or injured lung due to grief. I show two pathways: one direct and the other indirect.

Mother-son is the nurturing (strengthening direct relationship) outer clockwise arrow.

Grandfather-grandson is the controlling (supportive indirect relationship) inner arrow.

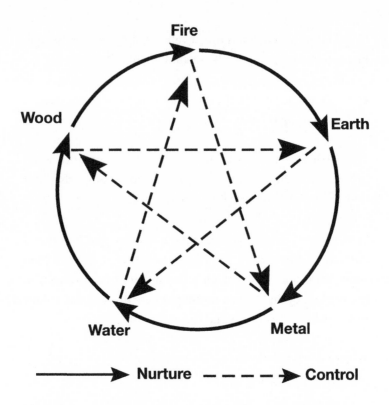

Example of imbalance of grandfather-grandson indirect relationship.

Here is an example of a poor diet causing the imbalance of grandfather-grandson indirect relationship. The earth or the nutrient chi affected the water chi with regard to my Sick Dad. I will start from my Sick Dad in his youth. He was active and full of life. Then over a slow process, he introduced himself to the junk things of life: soda, candy bars, ice cream, and comfort snacks. This affected his kidneys and was expressed with swelling of the legs in his later years.

That led to problems with his fire (heart) through the occurrences of four heart attacks, which caused him to be less active and made him retire to his recliner. This affected his metal (lung), and the last year of his life, he could no longer function without oxygen. He needed oxygen to sleep and to walk to the bathroom, which ultimately affected his wood (liver) with the inability to clean all the chemicals out of the body. That led to the earth (spleen) of only craving sugar for energy to more water retention or swelling of his body—the water (kidney). On May 22 at 4:40 p.m., he spent his last drop of the kidney chi. His heart had enough, and he took his last breath.

WHAT IS THE DIFFERENCE IN THE YIN TO YANG ORGANS?

The yin organs are the "essence" organs: heart, lung, liver, kidney, and pancreas. They produce a vital or essential fluid or chi for the body.

The yang organs are the "function" organs: small intestine, large intestine, bladder, gallbladder, and stomach. They are containers that hold the yin organ essences to perform a function for the body.

The stronger these organs are and the better they function, the healthier you are.

HOW DO THE TRUE YIN AND PURE YIN WITH THE TRUE YANG AND THE PURE YANG WORK WITH THE FIVE ELEMENTS?

After learning about yin-yang and the five element theory, I wanted to know how they both tie in together. My Healthy Dad went on to explain.

Earth is true yin; water is the pure yin; wood is the true yang; fire is the pure yang; metal/air is the balancer.

The balancer is the lung. This is where you get the air to burn the fire. In a classical sense, it is not yin or yang, but we know the lung is a yin or essence organ as the large intestine is a yang function organ. If you don't have enough oxygen, the heart struggles, your metabolic rate is affected, and you will not have the energy chi exchange.

One of the chi or energy sources from outside is the air; this is yin but enables yang fire. Wood makes the air and consumes the carbon dioxide, which is why aging is directly proportional to intercellular fluid balances.

Epigenetic chemicals are what ages the person from the injury to true yin (junk food, chemicals, and bad fats) that injures the strength of the liver, so the liver has to work overtime to clean the chemicals out of the body.

For example, when someone is detoxing, they may feel sicker because they are eliminating these chemicals from their body. This is why you do the daily detox nutrient "mix" (found in Chapter 6) to eliminate chemicals from the body.

When you have a dry lung (the balancer), you can have an injury to yin due to excess yang. In the case of excess yang, you create heat. In the case of excess yin, you create phlegm from the damp cold condition in the lung. In the principle of the five elements, the lung time is the fall season. It is the dry part of the year when you get seasonal colds and flu, and when you get a lung problem, it is because the lung needs to be slightly moist all the time. The principle is that if you don't have moisture, you can't absorb oxygen. If the alveoli becomes dry, you will have a fever syndrome due to dehydration of the lung or yang condition.

When you have a yin condition of the lung, you have too much moisture or dampness, resulting in pneumonia.

CONCLUSION

In this chapter, we learned that the five elements give you ways to determine what your nature is so you can understand how to apply these principles to create health. These are based on more than 4,000 years of **empirical knowledge** and have been used to create health in one-fourth of the world's population. Take the time to study this chapter for much greater depth of how natural elements affect the body and being.

What attitude element is more prevalent in you at this present moment?

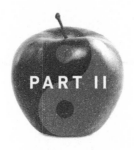

PART II

Primary Factors
of Health

CHAPTER 5

Eat for Your Health: Every Culture Has Its Culture

Did you know that your body is so dynamic that if given a pure quality lifestyle, especially in nutrition as well as motion, rest, energy, and love, it will produce its own probiotics to maintain and support your immune system?

Growing up, there were two signs that had a lasting imprint in my mind. I previously mentioned the sign in the school cafeteria when I was in elementary school which read, "You are what you eat." Then, in college, above the clock in the anatomy and physiology room, a sign said, "Time will pass. Will you?" Isn't it amazing how some phrases and signs stick with us? It is like a song played on the radio while you are driving to work. For some reason you cannot get rid of it; it's stuck in your head the rest of the day. I will discuss the first sign now and save the other one for later.

As I reflect on the meaning, "You are what you eat" is truer than ever. Let's dive into this chapter to see why what we eat has a direct correlation to our immune system. If there is ever a point and time in our life to understand what we eat, it is now!

WHAT ARE BENEFICIAL INTESTINAL BACTERIA?

It is said that the "nutrient chi sponsors the immune chi." In plain English, what does that mean? The better the quality of your food, the better your immune system functions. The better you can digest the food and have it mix well with the good bacteria, the more effectively the intestines will grow good bacteria. Eighty-five percent of your immune system is directly related to the beneficial bacteria in your gut (or intestinal tract). The good bacteria provide and create beneficial by-products the body needs.

1. Hydrogen peroxide, an antimicrobial, is one of those by-products.
2. B vitamins are created by the bacterial metabolism.
3. Gut bacteria breaks down the foods so the enzymes can transform it into nutrients that can then be absorbed into the blood.
4. Gut bacteria helps to bulk up and clump together the waste products so elimination will be more regular.

The more you have a bowel movement on a regular basis, the healthier your intestinal tract is.

If you do not have one to two regular bowel movements a day, then really pay attention to the change in your diet so you have regular eliminations daily. There are other issues that you may also look into, such as physical restrictions and emotional stresses, as these affect the elimination rhythm. If your intestines are good, you will be healthy.

Like in a compost pile, the bacteria break foods down into recyclable nutrients. Your intestine does this for you so that the nutrients are in a state that now enables the body's enzymes to change the nutrients so they can enter your bloodstream. There are beneficial bacteria on all the external membranes of the body, which is a critical factor in your health. It's like a force field that protects you. Knowing this, you may not want to use harsh chemicals and antibacterial soaps on your skin, as it will kill the good bacteria. These are clues to keeping healthy.

WHAT DO YOU MEAN BY HAVING YOUR OWN YOGURT FACTORY INSIDE OF YOU?

Healthy Dad told me I have a yogurt factory inside my body. This perplexed me, so I asked him about it. He explained that these bacteria in your intestines provide you with defense from other things growing in you that are not healthy for you. One main by-product of the bacteria growth is hydrogen peroxide. When it comes into contact with anaerobic bacteria, it will kill the bad bacteria as well as molds, yeasts, and fungus. Think of your intestinal tract as a yogurt factory. It ferments the food and puts out these by-products to aid your digestion, which keeps the intestine working better. This is the main support for your immune system—that is, the lung and large intestine connection.

IS THIS WHY I SEE SO MANY FUNGAL TOENAILS IN MY PRACTICE?

Yes. If you have extremely low good bacteria in your intestines, there is going to be a higher instance of yeast, molds, and fungi presented in your body. One of the first signs that your immune system is depleted can be seen by the yellowing and thick nails of your toenails. The toenails tell a lot about a person's health.

WHAT DO YOU MEAN BY "EVERY CULTURE HAS ITS OWN CULTURE"?

All around the world, humans have always had some form of bacteria in their diet from fermented foods that they have eaten regularly to maintain better health. If you spend enough time understanding each country, you will discover some form of good probiotics or good bacteria eaten regularly in their food sources.

Thus, the term, "Every culture has its own culture." In Germany, there is sauerkraut. Japan has miso, natto, and tamari. Scandinavian countries eat yogurt. Here in the United States and Canada, we eat pickles, and France has kefir. In Switzerland, they consume buttermilk from grass-fed cows. In China, they eat fermented vegetables. Koreans eat kimchi, Indonesians have tempeh, and Hawaiians have poi.

In modern society, everyone eats processed foods and chemicals. This will kill the good bacteria and create poor health which leads to diseases like diabetes, heart disease, autoimmune diseases, cancer, and most all modern ones. Remember, *food is your best medicine.*

WHAT ARE SOME FERMENTED FOODS AND PROBIOTICS?

The best source of good bacteria comes from homemade fermented vegetables and organic raw milk. Products like yogurt, kefir, lassi, or other cultured milk products are good sources. Additionally, there are fermented vegetables or foods that are cultured like sauerkraut, kimchi, and other pickled fermentations like cabbage, turnips, carrots, onions, and cucumbers. Some fermented soy foods (organic only) like miso, tamari, tempeh, and natto will also work.

IS THERE A PILL FORM OF PROBIOTICS?

If you are looking for a pill form, it is best to get one with 5–10 billion CFUs (colony-forming units) in a capsule that is refrigerated, and not off the shelf. It is good to have a multiple strains of bacteria in each capsule. Probiotics strain *lactobacillus acidophilus* is one of the best for general use. I like Green Vibrance as it has twelve kinds of probiotics and 25 billion CFUs per scoop, but there are other ones you may find from specialty vendors. Research these products and use them daily for better health. However, the active strains of bacteria in cultured foods are more potent than any bottle of acidophilus will ever be. Cultured foods are better.

Every thirty seconds bacteria double, so if you have an active strain fed good quality nutrients (called prebiotics) in balance, you will proliferate the bacteria quickly. In one minute, the bacteria would quadruple; in an hour, it would be 1,280 times the original amount. This will create billions of good bacteria in one hour. Thus, if you take an active culture with 100 billion beneficial bacteria in a tablespoon of quality fermented food, you will have consumed 10 trillion in an hour! Think of that. Now realize high-quality, freeze-dried capsules with a billion CFUs have only at best 3–5 percent bacteria that will cultivate, which is only 50 million after an hour. The cost of a capsule is far greater than a tablespoon of grass-fed yogurt. Yogurt has trillions of active bacteria per cup. There are approximately 100 trillion good bacteria in the gut of healthy people. Guard your good bacteria as your best friend!

Now you see what I mean when I say, *Chemistry is an assault on biology.* Chemicals, preservatives, and man-made things such as vitamins (chemistry) will harm the natural process of growing good bacteria in your body at the cellular level (biology).

CAN YOU TELL ME ABOUT THE OPTIMAL FACTORS THAT HELP THESE BACTERIA TO GROW IN OUR INTESTINES?

There are eight main principles to understanding how to grow good bacteria in your gut.

1. Time: It takes twelve hours for bacteria to grow.
2. Temperature: Bacteria prefer body temperature (98.6°).
3. Alkalinity: The ideal blood pH is 7.4.
4. Glucose: A good source for bacteria to grow on; whole grains are recommended, as you metabolize them more slowly.
5. Vegetables: For bulk, to help prevent compaction in the intestines.
6. Darkness: The intestine has no light.
7. Bacteria culture: Either fermented food or a capsule of acidolphilus, to introduce bacteria to your intestine.
8. Chyme: Liquefied food well-chewed twenty-five-plus times before swallowing.

WHAT HAPPENS IF YOUR BODY TEMPERATURE IS NOT AT 98.6°?

What happens when you're not 98.6°? You can't grow the right bacteria, and you're never healthy! What is the yin and yang factor? Yin is cold, and yang is hot. If you're below 98.6°, you're going to have a chronic immune problem. Why do I say 60–72 percent of all people need the immune diet in Chapter 9, which is based on the yangizing principle? Most people are too yin/cold and can't get their temperature up to grow the good bacteria. All people have to do is take their temperature. Their temperature will be below 98.6°. If they have a temperature above 98.6°–99.0°, they never get a cold, they never get the flu, they never get sick because they're more yang. They may have other problems like heart disease and diabetes if their lifestyle is poor, but they will not have sinus problems or digestive problems.

WHAT HAPPENS IF YOUR TEMPERATURE IS RUNNING HIGHER ON A DAILY BASIS WITHOUT FLU-LIKE SYMPTOMS OR YANG-DEFICIENCY SYNDROMES?

Over one hundred years ago, there were more yang people as the lifestyle was more physical and their diet was based on meats. Back in the 1850s–1900s, people would take an old-time remedy called the Jarvis remedy, which is apple cider vinegar and honey. This remedy will clean out gallbladder stones and alkalize the liver. This yang condition could take in more fluids, fruits, and vegetables to cool this higher temperature, and they got better.

From this principle, if your temperature is around 96°, your body will not produce the good bacteria your body needs. What if you're over 98.6°? Does that mean you're producing more bacteria, or are you too hot that you are now destroying the good bacteria? No, not until you have a fever of over 99.5°, which is when the body is ramping up in the immune system to fight off the yin condition. The optimal range of temperature for beneficial bacteria growth is in the 1° range of 98.2°–99.2°. The most important factor is to have quality prebiotics (nutrition) for the probiotics to grow on or they will not grow efficiently.

Have you ever heard the saying, "An apple a day keeps the doctor away?" Hint: Now you know why I used an apple with red yang and blue yin on the front cover of my book.

WHAT DID YOU MEAN BY HAVING A PH OF 7.4 IN THE BLOOD?

The pH level of your blood is 7.4. Anything below 7.0 is acid and this is toxic to the body. Over time, it will cause arthritis, cancer, and most illnesses. Anything over 7.4 is alkaline and will cause similar problems in the body. Both will make the body stiff and cause less inter-/extracellular transportation, which causes the cells to build up waste and lower the function of all the cells in the body. Between 7.2 and 7.4 blood pH is where the body will have less inflammation and irritation. One of the more beneficial reasons for being a vegetarian is to keep your body in an alkaline state. Do note that stress and toxic chemicals can be more acidifying than vegetables and fruits. It is important to know that deep breathing will alkalize you faster than food will.

WHAT DID YOU MEAN BY TWELVE HOURS TO PROCESS GOOD BACTERIA?

Bacteria will grow or incubate continuously on the food you eat through the digestive system, which takes about twelve hours to process foods before it gets to the end of the large intestine. A good probiotic with 5 billion CFU is almost as efficient as a fermented food because when it gets to the intestinal tract, it starts to propagate within minutes: 5 billion becomes 10 billion, which becomes 20 billion in minutes. But remember, at best, 5 percent will become active. One billion good bacteria as stated in the factors of optimal growing conditions double every thirty seconds. An active food strain will have 50–100 billion per tablespoon, so it will take only a few minutes to equal the 300 or 500 billion. The cost does not usually warrant the need to buy an expensive probiotic with 5 billion or higher CFU. A good commercial grass-fed cow's yogurt is better and less expensive as it has 50–100 billion per tablespoon or even more when it is homemade.

WHEN DO YOU GET YOUR FIRST BACTERIA INTRODUCED TO START YOUR IMMUNE SYSTEM?

Here is a subject that has not really been talked about much, but I feel it is so important to be addressed. The baby inoculation of the mother's bacteria, by way of vaginal birth, is better understood by saying "the mother's vaginal inoculation." When a child is born, their first inoculation or "natural vaccination" occurs when the mother is having a normal birth, and the head crowns and the lips of the baby now touch the vaginal wall of the mother. It is the first exposure of a foreign substance to the child. During the first three days of breastfeeding, colostrum is introduced into the baby. This colostrum is the best prebiotic and will kill any bacteria that are not of the inherited bacteria from the mother. It has immunosuppressive properties that will only allow her strain of bacteria to grow, no other one, good or bad. This becomes the resident strain for life. This is the very first step to your immune system being developed. It is the first defense for your health. If you do not get this bacterium at birth, you will have health issues your whole life because immunity starts in the digestive system.

IS THERE ANY RECOMMENDATION IF A CHILD HAS TO BE DELIVERED BY CESAREAN?

Yes, it is my recommendation that when the child is born, the doctor swabs the vagina and places it on the lips of the baby. It sounds off the wall, but you have to remember, a normal birth is a natural birth where we are born by coming out of the vaginal canal. Now, there is a problem with this technique of the swab inoculation; if the mother has been given antibiotics just before birth, it will kill the good bacteria in the mother. That means there is no starter bacteria on the swab. Sorry to say this, but now the new baby has a big consequence to overcome. There is a reason for this, and it's not talked about at all. It's the inoculation. It is also important to start breastfeeding the baby to get the colostrum that will give the baby the natural anti-foreign microbial suppressive nutrients to start its life.

ARE THERE OTHER FACTORS THAT PLAY INTO THE HEALTH OF A BABY?

There are other factors that will come into play, such as emotional issues and the brain function if the mother was eating healthy during her pregnancy. But remember, a natural vaginal birth is the most important factor.

CAN YOU EXPLAIN TO ME WHY GLUCOSE IS NEEDED TO CREATE GOOD BACTERIA?

Getting back on track with optimal growing factors, I had to proceed to ask the question, because in my mind, sugar is not good for the body, and most people who are aware of their health refrain from sugars. What did you mean when you said glucose is needed to create good bacteria? I meant that the glucose that comes from organic grains is the best form of sugar. It is a primary factor needed in the bacterial growing environment. This is why I use short-grain brown rice because it's one of the best foods to eat. All grains are carbohydrates (complex sugars), which become glucose, which is an important nutrient (prebiotic) for the bacteria to grow on. Carbohydrates are important to the body for energy, which creates heat, yang, thus it maintains your temperature! If you sit on a couch after eating and don't utilize the carbohydrate, it becomes a fat called triglyceride.

If that fat cell's main purpose is excessive fuel storage, the carbohydrates now sit around in a fat cell for a long duration. The fat cells become a storage container for toxic chemicals. To get them out of the blood, think what it's like sweeping dirt under a rug when you didn't have time to pick it up and get rid of it. Inorganic chemicals (man-made) cause cancer by interfering in the DNA communications with the RNA, which is done through a chemical language, so to speak. The toxic epigenetic chemicals are what they are called. When you use the simple sugars that come from a good source such as grains, it can aid in the process of optimal bacteria formation in the intestines.

After thinking about what I heard, this is how I applied this information and what I observed. Reflecting on my experience with my Sick Dad, after dinner was done, we would be back outside working until the sun went down. All those carbohydrates from the potatoes and bread were utilized and put into energy. They were really never stored up as fat cells. Mild exercise or activity after eating helps digestion. Maybe this is why I continued to exercise after my dinner throughout college and my current career.

WHY IS CHEWING YOUR FOODS SO IMPORTANT?

The longer you chew your food, the more the carbohydrate will break down before it gets into the stomach, as amylase (starch enzyme) in the saliva is secreted in the mouth to start the breaking-down process. It is recommended that you chew your food at least twenty-five-plus times before swallowing. Toasting your bread will dry it out, so you will chew it better, you will chew more, and that makes it more easily hydrated with the saliva. The saliva has amylase, which starts to work on grains to turn carbohydrates into glucose. When you chew longer, it will break down better. So now your bacteria will work on it and ferment it as it travels through the digestive system. If you don't have the good bacteria and the correct temperature, you'll ferment it into bad bacteria. This will give you more gas and digestive troubles.

Healthy Dad gave an example to explain what he had just told me, about a man who was in the army and stationed in Japan when a bomb went off and large amounts of radiation were released that caused the good bacteria to be killed in his intestinal lining. He never drank alcohol, but for some reason, he got a specific kind of yeast infection due to the radiation he was exposed to. So when he ate any sugar or carbohydrates, he got drunk because it fermented inside of him.

When he came home from the war, he got a job and he would eat regular food with grain in it, like a sandwich. He would get drunk. This *drunken* phenomenon went on for twenty-five years. He would always get drunk when he ate and yet he never drank any alcohol. He was labeled an alcoholic, and he lost every job shortly after getting hired. Then he lost his wife, he lost his house, he lost everything.

After reading about a doctor in Japan who was treating the condition he had, he went back to Japan and was treated by this doctor. He was treated by ingesting fermented garlic, and he recovered completely. Upon returning home, his life returned back to normal and he never got drunk from eating foods that had sugar or carbohydrates in them. This is what happens in the intestinal tract when you don't have good microbes.

In this example, the radiation killed all the good and bad microbes as well as yeast and molds, so he was like a newborn baby having no microbes in the intestine. His first inoculation must have been a yeast-like beer that causes the carbohydrates in food to ferment into alcohol in his digestive tract. Yes, it is an extreme case, but it is real.

I would think twice about starting a diet that didn't have you eat any grains. When I say grains, it is my recommendation to use organic brown rice as you like. I use organic Lundberg short-grain brown rice as it has fewer chemicals in it. This is a good source of sugar to aid in the making of beneficial bacteria. Make sure you're buying organic grains because you don't want grains containing chemicals that will affect the growth of beneficial bacteria.

CAN YOU EXPLAIN HOW A FREEZE-DRIED PROBIOTIC WORKS?

What happens is, if you take an acidophilus capsule or probiotic, it has 5 billion freeze-dried active units in it, and you may get only 3 percent that will cultivate. This means only some will wake up and become alive, and the other 97 percent will never return to life due to the drying process and time it takes to get the units from production to consumption. When you have a good source of a medium, such as sugar that comes from an organic source, the probiotic will now have a base where it can multiply and be more productive. In a normal situation, only 2–3 percent is acidophilus and 90–95 percent is sugar, which is FOS (a form of rice sugar).

A good strain will have up to 3–5 percent, and a bad strain will have as little as 1 percent. Those found on the shelf and not refrigerated will have this percentage. The ones in the refrigerator have more, the ones with dry space do better, and the ones that are freeze-dried are even better. If you have one that is already active, it is much more efficient! The take-home message is that the better quality of probiotic in a combination of a good organic source of grain sugar like brown rice or whole wheat and rolled oats will provide the medium for the most optimal way to grow good bacteria in your body!

WHICH IS BETTER—YOGURT OR A VEGETABLE PROBIOTIC LIKE SAUERKRAUT?

Which is more active? Grass-fed yogurt or sauerkraut? You'll do better with yogurt because it's a lactobacillus, which is closer to mother's milk. It is more digestible and most people are inclined to eat dairy rather than vegetables. Yogurt is the perfect formula for milk glucose and lactose. The lactose in the milk is what the bacteria attach to or grow on, and glucose aids in the process of helping it grow. Consider lactobacillus in the grass-fed yogurt that contains about 5 billion active bacteria per tablespoon. About one teaspoon will grow to 1 trillion in a quarter cup as long as it has its optimal growth factors: temperature of 98.4°, pH of 7.4, dark environments, twelve hours, and a good source of medium or sugar.

The main point I make here is having just one teaspoon of yogurt from a quality organic farm that has grass-fed cows, and not grain-fed cows, is better than a whole bottle of acidophilus or what you buy at the grocery store. It is even better than freeze-dried products. It is a live bacterium. It will be a hundred times more active. When this happens, the bacteria double every thirty seconds. It multiplies by four in the first minute, so you know you have four times as much in one minute than you did before you started. Just do the math. After an hour, you will have over a trillion.

WHAT IS THE MAIN THING THAT IS HURTING OUR IMMUNE SYSTEM?

The main thing that is hurting our immune system (via our good bacteria) is chemicals, especially glyphosate and antibiotics. Glyphosate is "Roundup," which is patented as an antimicrobial. It is the chemical used to spray weeds to kill them! Because it is water soluble, it can be found in our water, air, and also the soil where it was sprayed. You will learn more about this in the chapter on the quality of our foods.

What does it mean to be lactose intolerant?

Lactose intolerant people are sensitive to casein, a milk protein. These people are usually the ones who do not have good bacteria because they were exposed to toxic chemicals, Roundup, antibiotics, hormones, and steroids at a very young age. They got earaches or ingrown toenails and were placed on antibiotics. They were exposed to glyphosate in their foods. They drank milk that contained hormones and steroids with chemicals like Roundup (glyphosate) in it. And some infants were given baby formula instead of their mother's breast milk. All these things killed off their good microbes.

Humans are designed to digest lactose. Why are they not able to? Because they didn't get their starter culture from their mother. Due to the circumstances of the mother, they were born with a C-section and/or they were bottle-fed with baby formula and never breastfed. Now you can understand the bacterial principle and you'll learn why an immune diet will address this condition. The immune diet is nothing more than giving you the balance of yin and yang in your food, and the temperature will help to make the good bacteria grow. That's why it's based on chicken, rice, vegetables, alkalinity, warmth, and glucose. That's the principle of the immune diet.

CONCLUSION

Treat the body the way it was intended to be treated by nature and it will serve you well. We literally are what we eat. When you eat to survive or to socialize, be more observant of the foods you are eating. As you do this, you will be on the right path to good health. I wonder if my Sick Dad would have had a better retirement if he had eaten a little better and established good bacteria on a daily basis. What I did notice from my Healthy Dad was this was the main staple in his daily routine. He knew if he established a good environment with the right temperature and good medium of a quality sugar, such as an organic rolled oats or organic brown rice, his body would produce good bacteria to keep him healthy, free from any medications, illness, and diseases. At seventy years old, my Healthy Dad is very active and in good health without any medical drugs or major health conditions. So this lifestyle must be healthy!

What is your body temperature? Are you eating foods that will give you the yogurt factory your body needs to produce good bacteria? What is the one thing today that you can avoid eating or drinking?

CHAPTER 6

Basic Nutritional Concepts: Quality versus Non-quality

The main food pyramid recommends eating fruits and vegetables, proteins, grains, and fats, but nothing is said about the quality of each item. Could you be setting the course for ailments and illness in the future by eating what you think is good for you by following the recommended charts without knowing they have chemicals in them?

WHAT DO I MEAN BY QUALITY WITH REGARD TO FOOD AND WATER/FLUIDS?

I often hear from one who is dieting, "I am eating really well" and "I am on this vegan diet." Or "I am on this keto diet." I then follow up with a question: "How do you feel?" They respond, "I feel great!" Six months later, I will ask again how they feel. "I feel good, but my energy is down. Why am I sluggish?" I will ask when you follow the diets, "Do you look at the type and quality of foods you're eating, or do you just buy the food that is recommended and eat it?"

Do not underestimate the simple word "quality." I want you to observe those friends of yours who have been on diets, and ask yourself why is it that they follow a diet and they seem to get better initially only to find themselves off their diet and searching for a new one?

The answer is very simple. Almost all diets have a short shelf life. A diet does not address the person on an individual basis. Diets can be either too yin (vegan, fruit-only diets), or they can be yang (Atkins or keto). At some point, the body just says, "Hey, wait a minute. Time out! I think you should rethink this way of eating!" Or it may tell you, "You are feeding me all these good things, but why am I not feeling good?" The answer boils down to these simple principles: the five elements, yin and yang, and chemical-free quality.

I will touch upon the quality of water, air, foods, and minerals in this chapter to help you better understand the importance of quality. There are three physical sustenances our human body needs to survive and thrive: air, water, and food (nutrition). We will talk about three nonphysical sustenances you need later: love, community, and purpose. In these physical elements, quality is the key factor! Healthy Dad would often repeat himself on such matters. Over time, I started to pay attention to these areas. When I was not asking questions, he would always repeat something that we had just discussed. He always repeated quality of food, water, and air.

WHAT IS THE BEST WATER OUT THERE TO DRINK?

Healthy Dad would always say, "Know what is *not* in your water!" If I know what is not in my water (or have pure water), then I can always add what is needed. Reverse osmosis (RO) water is the best and here is why: I would rather know what is in my water than assuming that it is good. Yes, RO takes all the minerals out of the water and it becomes acidic, which becomes toxic to our body. This is why I add ConcenTrace "trace minerals" back into the water so I know what is in the water I am drinking. These minerals will alkalize the water. ConcenTrace liquid sea minerals are in an ionic state, which is the type that is in your blood, so this is the easiest form of minerals to absorb. One of those mineral elements is iodine, which is very hard to get in foods. The purest form of water is the body's best friend. Adding these sea minerals helps at the cellular level with the inter-/extracellular transportation, which adds to the elimination of toxic metals and chemicals.

Minerals help with cellular respiration (inter-/extracellular transportation), which can facilitate the elimination of fluorides, chlorine, Roundup, hormones, steroids, antibiotics, heavy metals, and phosphates. This can be accomplished by adding fifteen to twenty drops of ConcenTrace to a quart of water, which is my recommendation for most people if done two times a day. ConcenTrace provides a mineral balance in the blood plasma that will create an osmotic pressure causing an isotonic balance, thus liberating the intercellular toxins. As a liquid desalinated sea water, ConcenTrace also alkalizes the water. You can also create energized water by putting it in a round glass jug and stirring it clockwise for a minute and then refrigerating it.

HOW DO I KNOW IF I HAVE TOO MUCH OR TOO LITTLE WATER IN MY SYSTEM?

Have a minimum of two quarts of quality fluids a day. Did you notice I said quality fluids? Every place is different. In the desert, you will need more water than in a cooler climate. No matter where I live, I will always look at my urine. Yes, it sounds gross, but here is the truth in what I am saying. If your urine is too clear, then you're getting too much water, or you are too yin. Clear urine will overload your kidneys by unnecessarily making them work harder. If your urine is too dark (a deeper yellow), then you are too yang. In extreme cases, it will have an orange tint, which means you are not getting enough fluids and you will need more.

Healthy Dad said, "Compare your urine to light beer." I asked, "Beer? I have never had a beer. I was always the designated driver!" But your urine can be that color even without beer! Ha! He explained, "We need a light coloration in our urine. Just know it is best to have just a bit of color to the urine for good hydration of the body cells and to not deplete your blood plasma of the minerals you need. Watch the urine. If it has too much color all day, you will need to drink more fluids, but if the urine is clear in the morning, then drink less that day. So each time you urinate, you can determine how much you need to hydrate. Just know **WATER** = **hydration** and **hydration is the best anti-inflammatory.**

WHAT CAN YOU TELL ME ABOUT REVERSE OSMOSIS AND DISTILLED WATER?

Distilled water is water that is acidic and free of dissolved minerals. It has the ability to wash out toxic substances from the body for elimination. It's kind of like RO but in a different process. People will use these to detoxify their bodies and it may be helpful for a week or two. But without minerals, it will deplete you and not work as well as a detoxifier. The downside is, the longer you drink it, the more likely you will develop mineral deficiencies and form an acidic state. Some of the side effects are cardiac irregularities, high blood pressure, and cognitive and emotional disturbances.

Healthy Dad explained RO and distilled is where you take everything out and "now you know what's NOT in your water." If you add the ConcenTrace minerals back into it, this will bring the pH value to more alkaline levels. RO is a much easier and cheaper means to getting pure water, which is why I use RO. Remember, the first thing you want to do in the morning is hydrate yourself with fluid.

When you first wake up, you've had an eight-hour period of time when you didn't drink anything, so you're a little bit dehydrated. In the morning, look at the color of your urine, and it will tend to be darker than during the day. You want to hydrate with minerals in the fluids so you replenish your electrolytes in the blood. Proper hydration is important as this will allow for more plasma, which thins the blood. You want to drink something warming for the stomach if you are too yin and you want to have something purifying for the liver and to increase the fluid for the intestine. Dehydration causes constipation. You absorb your fluids in the large intestine. If you don't have enough fluid, you're going to have constipation from dehydration because you're going to absorb the fluid that's in the intestinal tract to maintain the blood plasma hydration.

It is important to keep your blood plasma at a certain level of hydration. The most important thing you can do first thing in the morning is to drink something and wait thirty minutes before you eat. I put trace minerals in my water because I want to hydrate. I want to take the minerals in the ConcenTrace because that facilitates getting the fluid into the cell, not just into the blood. You are going to have a stronger day because of your ability to maintain intercellular fluid inside the cells. That's how your muscle cells maintain their tone. If you don't have enough minerals, you can't keep that fluid in the muscle cell, which results in weak muscles.

WHY DO I USE CONCENTRACE LIQUID SEA MINERALS IN THE MORNING?

Because ConcenTrace has all the trace minerals in a liquid ionic state the way the blood plasma needs them. I want to hydrate the cells so those minerals can get into my cells.

WHAT IS THE BEST BEVERAGE I CAN TAKE TO START MY DAY?

The best beverage to drink in the morning is the daily Detox Nutrient Mix to nourish and detox your blood and clean the intestine, liver, and tissue cells of heavy metals and chemical toxins. It is best to take it an hour before eating anything. This way, it gets into the blood faster and goes straight to the liver to hydrate and clean it. It is good to have a second one late afternoon if you choose to. For convenience, it is good to premix the dry bulk products and create your own premade container of the mix. Do it in a ratio close to the ingredients listed below. Put the RO water in a glass jar, add the ConcenTrace liquid sea water, and if you like, add a tart fruit juice, and then add your tablespoon or more of the mix. Now put the lid on and shake it well to mix thoroughly. When you do this in this order, then you won't have clumps that stick to the bottom of the jar.

WHAT IS IN THE DAILY DETOX NUTRIENT MIX?

- ½ tsp of spirulina powder, a complete protein, B vitamin, and chlorophyll concentration
- ¼ tsp of sodium alginate powder
- ¼ tsp of red marine algae powder
- ¼ tsp apple or fruit pectin powder
- 1 tsp psyllium husk powder for bulk, so adjust to your needs
- 25–40 drops of ConcenTrace, which is liquid seawater for trace minerals (this is not in the premix so you will have to add it)

NOTE: If your stools are too loose, then back off to half of the number of liquid drops. You may want to start lower at first like fifteen to twenty drops and work your way up to a comfortable level.

OTHER ITEMS YOU WILL BE ADDING TO THE MIXTURE IN ADDITION TO WHAT WAS JUST MENTIONED

One-half teaspoon of Green Vibrance. It has probiotics and sixty freeze-dried organic veggies and herbs. This too is not added in the mixture, so you can add it separately. It is not necessary, but it's good. You may choose to flavor the beverage by using any of these tart fruit juices: cherry, cranberry, blueberry, pomegranate, or any berries liquid juice or concentrate to add to twelve ounces of RO water, which is the liquid for the mix. Use approximately two ounces of juice or one-half ounce of concentrated juice. Be sure these juices are not sweetened with any sweet fruit juice or artificial sugar. Another good option is to add the mix to a blend of 50 percent fresh vegetable juice to 50 percent RO water.

If you want to make it a bit more practical, you can take the following ingredients and make a bulk amount and keep it in the freezer. This way, you don't have to divide it out every day. Just get a large bowl and put the ingredients in and mix it very well. Here is how you divide up the ingredients for bulk storage use:

- 1 cup sodium alginate
- 1 cup red marine algae
- 1 cup apple or fruit pectin
- 2 cups psyllium
- 3 cups spirulina
- 3 cups Green Vibrance

I can't emphasize this enough to use RO H_2O, reverse osmosis water, so you know you do not have any chemicals or impurities in the water. DO NOT USE TAP WATER as it has bad chemicals, drugs, metals, chlorine, and fluoride in it. I've used this morning beverage for thirty years. It makes you bright-eyed and bushy-tailed! It also gives you almost a complete balance of nutrients from the spirulina and liquid sea minerals. Spirulina is very high in protein, but you'll also need omega-3 oils in the form of krill oil (750–1,000 mg). This gives you a nutritive boost to the liver and blood plasma, and the fats from the omega-3 oils go to the liver and make the bad fats metabolize. That's why I'll take the krill oil separately and then I'll take the mix that consists of the spirulina, the liquid sea minerals, and seaweeds, and then the bulking agent. Sodium alginate is a seaweed. The apple pectin and psyllium are bulking agents, so that's going to hydrate and bulk up the large intestine and facilitate the bacteria growth. It will bond your toxicity to the intestinal tract material to elim-inate it. Eighty-five percent of the toxins never get into your blood because the bacteria in your intestine bind these toxins and attach them to the cellulose fibers in your intestinal tract and carry them all out in the stool. The toxins never even go to the liver. This morning beverage is the most purifying and nourishing thing you can do.

If you do this mix every morning, you'll get more nutrition than most people get in a week even if they eat well!

CAN YOU TELL ME MORE ABOUT THE DAILY DETOX NUTRIENT MIX?

1. Good minerals will create an osmotic potential to exchange the bad products out of the cells to be eliminated and get the good products into the cell for proper hydration and nutrition. This is called cellular respiration. The products in the mix are high in trace minerals; iodine and magnesium are especially important as most people are deficient in these minerals. Also have seaweed, seawater, seafood, and marine algae generally in your diet.

2. Spirulina and red algae are great chlorophylls. Most people think green when you say chlorophyll, but you need a full color spectrum—blue, red, orange, and yellow—to give you a variety of chlorophylls that are not talked about much but are necessary in your diet. You will also get a good amount of calcium and magnesium, which will create an alkalinity in the blood that will help the osmotic transportation of the cells. Spirulina also has a very good amount of quality protein and some vitamin C. It is also good to eat up to two cups of lightly cooked greens a day—kale, collards, and cilantro or other greens—to give you some fresher types of chlorophyll depending on your yin-yang nature.

3. Omega-3 oils (especially DHA) are essential to your health and will increase immunity by elevating your vitamin D3 (now called the immune hormone), which helps calcium absorption, which, in turn, increases the pH to alkalize the

blood. Omega-3 oils will also increase your metabolic rate and act like a detergent to break down omega-6 LDL and omega-9 trans fats, which are the places where toxic chemicals and heavy metals are stored in the body. Take at least 750–1,000 mg of krill oil (or more) a day. Also, take one to two tablespoons of 100-percent grass-fed butter or add other quality fats to your diet.

4. Psyllium and apple or fruit pectin will suspend or bind the heavy metals and transport them out of your body. Pectin: Use 500 mg two times a day for each one hundred pounds of your body weight.

5. Good bacteria in probiotics and fermented foods and beverages will help the gut become healthier and will help immunity by providing the microbial action in the intestines for better digestion. This, along with roughage, will bind heavy metals in the foods and eliminate them in the stool. Take a variety of types of good bacteria multiple times a day.

6. Quality beverages will give you fluids that will help to eliminate the bad minerals. Drink RO H_2O in herb teas and drink green vegetable juices. Use enough to keep your urine almost clear with a tint of yellow, so drink more than you usually do and watch the color of your urine.

RO water will give you knowledge *TO KNOW WHAT IS NOT IN YOUR WATER!* RO water will provide you with fluid that contains none of the following:

1. Toxins: endocrine disruptors (hormones), steroids, antibiotics, glyphosate, genetically modified organisms (GMOs), and toxic heavy metals from industrial pollution such as geo-engineering also known as chemtrails: mercury, aluminum, nickel, cadmium, chromium, lead, cesium, barium, strontium.

2. Chemicals and pollution: pesticides, herbicides, drugs, fluoride and chlorine, polychlorinated biphenyl (PCB), and polymerizing vinyl chloride (PVC).
3. Particles larger than .5 microns: bacteria, amoebas, protozoa, and most viruses.

Other things you can do to increase the elimination of toxins:

1. Saunas and ionic foot baths help to detox heavy metals.
2. Exercise to perspire for more elimination.
3. Generally, eat good quality organic food properly prepared for your yin-yang nature.

HOW SOON CAN I EAT AFTER I DO THE DAILY DETOX NUTRIENT MIX IN THE MORNING?

It is best to wait for an hour before eating anything so the pure nutrients and fluids get into the blood before you eat. It affects the liver better as food slows its absorption. It is one of the safest detoxes that you can do, and you can do it all year round, seven days a week.

IS THIS SAFE FOR SOMEONE WHO IS PREGNANT?

Yes, but start with one-fourth the amount as you do not want to detox too fast. The ingredients are all-natural foods with good sources of minerals. I would even say to a pregnant woman, it is vital to have a good source of minerals in your body along with the good bacteria. The caution here is to take only one-fourth of the dose if you are not eating real good food during your pregnancy. If you take more, you will detox too fast and you'll have more nausea. Also, you don't want the baby to have more than it should have. As mentioned before, where does our first inoculation start? Yes, when the child comes down the birth canal and its lips touch the wall of the vaginal canal. Then in combination with breastfeeding, the child gets the colostrum in the first three days. That child will be set for the rest of his or her life. The mix will provide you and the baby with much better nutrition, so it will benefit the baby.

WHAT CAN YOU TELL ME IN REGARD TO THE QUALITY OF FOOD?

You can't put a price on your health! This is key to having a healthy life. You will want to find the best quality food: organic, locally grown in quality soil, seasonal, fresh, unprocessed, without chemicals or additives, and whole as nature built it.

Food is very important just as is the quality of water. Most of the illnesses and ailments that we face later in life will be directly correlated back to what we ate in our younger years. Most diets have good intentions, but very few of them are specific as to the quality of the foods. They will say no meats, or all vegetables, but they'll leave out the vital information. What is the key and most vital information? Eat real quality food! The fewer hands it took to get the food to your dinner table, the better off you will be.

Reflecting on this statement caused me to think about the conversations I've had with patients. They will present me with a question by stating, "I'm on a diet and eating better, but why am I not feeling any better?" Or, "Why is it that after a period of time I am back to where I began?" It does come down to the quality of the food you are eating. My advice is to keep it simple. If you're going to eat meat, then make sure it is grass-fed beef, free-range chicken, and wild-caught fish. If you're going to eat vegetables and fruits, then make sure they are organic as there is less exposure to chemicals. Because the quality of our soil is not like it used to be, we lack minerals in our soil which means less nutritional value to our biology (every cell in our body).

We are not getting the nutritional value out of our foods, so we remain hungry after eating. Here's a classic example. Go out to eat at your favorite fast-food place and order a hamburger, fries, and a soda. How do you feel after you are done eating? Are you still feeling empty inside and hungry? Well, the nutritional value of what you just ate is basically the same as the cardboard it was served in!

Your body is designed to function in a way that takes all the nutrients and uses them, but if there are no nutrients in your food, then you need more food to compensate for the deficiencies. Obesity is one of the most alarming conditions in America today. We are eating more not even knowing it because we need more quality nutrients in our foods and then you add this with a lack of exercise and being locked up in our homes causes more weight to be added to our body frame. It is time to wake up and realize what we are doing to our bodies!

WHY IS QUALITY OF FATS SO IMPORTANT?

When you have a good quality of fat, which is omega-3s, you have no need for insulin, so you circumvent that inflammation. You now have a higher vitamin D content, so you absorb your calcium. You have a stable pH in your body and now you can grow your beneficial bacteria. The bacteria is the main factor in breaking down your food to get the nutrition so the enzyme works on it. This is where you get your nutrition. The good fats go in and metabolize the bad fats.

Chemicals and heavy metals in your body (aluminum, mercury,

and glyphosate) accumulate in the dormant fat cells. When the fat tissue (adipose tissue) gets overloaded with these toxic chemicals and metals, they leach to the adjacent organ tissues, and this is the primary cause of cancer. If you don't have the good fats, you don't have the ability to break down the bad fats to mobilize the toxic material to eliminate them.

The main concept is, with omega-3 fats and trace minerals, especially iodine, you will raise your metabolic rate in the brain, which elevates your serotonin and endorphin levels (happy chemicals). Elevating these happy chemicals will increase the biological (body) metabolism, and you will then burn the stored bad fats for fuel. This puts the toxic chemicals back into the blood, which will enable them to be removed with the daily nutrient detox mix. This mix is one of the most natural ways to help remove the disease-causing toxins from your body.

Healthy Dad reiterated the truth of the statement, "You are what you eat." It is spot-on! Just by having a bowel movement does not mean you eliminate all the bad things you just consumed. "You want to eat good shit, man!" LOL! Ha! Yes, my Healthy Dad has a sense of humor.

WHAT ARE THE GOOD FATS?

Good quality fats are omega-3 fats (PUFA—polyunsaturated fatty acids) such as DHA, EPA, and ALA. These come from sources such as grass-fed meats and milk fats, butter, wild fish oils especially krill and salmon, all animals raised naturally along with free-range chicken and eggs. When you get these fats from your foods, you speed up the fat metabolism. Now when you add seawater (ConcenTrace), your body can do the cellular respiration better to get those heavy metals out of your cells. The apple pectin can bind the metals and transport them to the kidneys, hair, skin, and nails so you can eliminate the toxic metals. Do you see how all this works together with quality fats?

WHAT OTHER BENEFITS DO GOOD FATS HAVE?

I asked my Healthy Dad if we need vitamin D3 to process omega-3 oils. He would say, "No!" You need omega-3 oils to provide you with vitamin D if you do not get enough sunlight. Vitamin D will cause you to absorb calcium to make the body more alkaline, raise your body temp, and grow the good bacteria to create natural health.

By having a good quality of vitamin D3 in your system, this causes a higher amount of alkalinity in the body, which will help you produce calcium to maintain a calcium balance and the alkalinity in your blood. This helps you maintain alkalinity in your intestinal tract, which helps you to grow the right bacteria. What will help you produce your immune response? Good fats aid in the ability to produce vitamin D, which leads to a better immune system. The best sources of omega-3 fats to help you produce vitamin D3 aside from sunlight are from red krill oil, wild-caught salmon, grass-fed cow butter and fats, and free-range eggs.

WHAT STUDIES HAVE BEEN DONE THAT GIVE IMPORTANT INFORMATION ABOUT THE QUALITY OF OMEGA-3 FATS (DHA AND VITAMIN D)?

Weston A. Price, a dentist back in the early 1920s, traveled all over the world looking at people's teeth. His 528-page book *Nutrition and Physical Degeneration* expressed his research as he visited countries from all over the world. As I started to read his book, I became more fascinated at the information on pages twenty-two to twenty-five. He described the Loetschental Valley in the high Alpines of Switzerland. Here was a place he described as having no dentist, no physician, no policeman, and no jail because there was no need for them. Dr. Price also pointed out that the Vatican in Rome selected men from this valley to help guard the Vatican. Why? Because they were healthy, free from tuberculosis and other diseases in the world. They had very good immune systems. They would take the milk that was produced from the grass-fed cattle in early spring and make the butter. They would even have a worship program to welcome this early spring butter and cheese. This was vital because it was this milk that the cows produced after eating the fresh spring grasses. It was the highest quality, creating the richest milk fat of the year. It was this high quality of fat that came from the cow's milk in the spring that gave this village the nutrients to live a healthy and happy life, which they were reverent to.

The village elders would collect the milk fat and make butter to store for the community. Everyone would receive a small amount a day for the whole year as a supplement. This was so critical in their health that it became part of their belief system. Just like the Kosher laws and religious food rituals, all food customs are developed to keep people healthy. Then they become part of the religion, not the other way around! This was pointed out by Dr. Price in 1931–32 when he visited the village.

As I read more, I started to understand more. I was convinced my Sick Dad understood land, soil, and crops. I realized why I got in trouble when my father sent me down to the stackyard where all the hay was stored. He gave me specific instructions on what hay to sell and what hay was to be used for our cows. He was a little upset with me when he learned that I had sold the first-crop hay, when I should have sold the second-crop hay (still a quality hay but not like the first crop). If only my Sick Dad would have understood nutrition like he did crop rotation and how to raise animals, like the differences between the first-crop and the fourth-crop hay in his own diet, maybe he would have laid off the junk foods more. I am under my own impression that there are many "Swiss Valley" healthy communities all around us; we just don't know about them. To me, they are more priceless than gold mines. You can eat quality foods, but you can't eat a bar of gold. But one will say, "With the gold, I can buy more food!" Yes, you have a point there, but if there is no good food to buy, what good is your gold?

WHAT ABOUT THE QUALITY OF AIR?

"Prana chi" or "lung chi" respiration is the oxygen you take in from the air into your lungs; then you expel carbon dioxide out of the lungs. This is similar to the transfer of inter-/extracellular nutrients of the cells, so we will call it cellular respiration. In goes the good and out comes the bad. This is another way your body eliminates waste. This type of lung chi goes with a pace of life and rest to guard the kidney chi. Rhythmic breathing, which you do best in a deep sleep, has been an ancient practice to manage your vitality and emotions. It is a discipline that overrides the mind, so it is used in most spiritual practices. A good way to relax in times that are very stressful is to breathe in and then breathe out twice as long as you breathed in with a pause between the in and out. This will make your body less toxic or less acidic. It is important to realize you can alkalize your blood faster by deep breathing than you can by eating the highest quality alkaline food or beverages!

HAVE YOU EVER SEEN PLACES THAT ARE SO POLLUTED THAT THERE ARE MAJOR RESPIRATORY PROBLEMS?

Yes, most major cities in the world have air quality issues and can cause respiratory issues for people. So if you live in a major city, you are not doomed, but you really need to follow what I am saying with the quality of foods and waters. This will help to eliminate pollutants from your body. Also grow indoor green plants. The more you grow, the better that air will be.

IS THERE A PROPER WAY TO BREATHE?

One simple way to breathe is to put one hand on your chest and one hand on your abdomen, and watch which hand goes up. If the hand on your chest goes up, you need to change your breathing. You need to see the hand on your abdomen go up. This is the proper way to breathe because it activates the abdomen organs. This motion will pump these organs, and you will get more circulation, which increases their function. I will also mention that taking in a deep breath or deep breathing is important in so many ways. It is simple. Just breathe in deep and breathe out twice as long as you breathe in, especially when you encounter something that is really stressful.

I replied by telling my Healthy Dad about a fascinating book by Eckhart Tolle called *The Power of Now*. Eckhart mentions in his book that you can't think and breathe at the same time. Therefore, when you focus on your breath, it brings you to the present moment so you are not worrying about the future things of life that do not exist. Healthy Dad agreed, explaining that stress is even more damaging to the body than most bad foods because it lowers your immune system. Breathing properly to release stress has an emotional component to helping our immune system, along with the quality of our foods, water, and air we breathe.

HOW I APPLIED THIS PRINCIPLE OF PROPER BREATHING IN MY PRACTICE

Have you ever wondered why it is so hard for someone to quit smoking? It is because they are addicted to breathing! Smokers know how to breathe properly! When they become stressed, they grab the cigarette and start to smoke. This allows them to breathe properly; they will breathe in the smoke and breathe out twice as long to get the smoke out. When they do this, it starts to relax their mind and body. It makes their body less acidic. So if you want to quit smoking, learn how to breathe without the cigarette and you can quit smoking. The best way to quit smoking is when you are stressed and you grab the cigarette, just don't light it. Instead, put the cigarette in your mouth and pretend to smoke, learn how to breathe properly without the cigarette. Eventually you will quit smoking because now you know how to relax without the need for the cigarette. I have had many patients of mine quit smoking by just using this simple principle.

WHAT IS CHELATION, AND HOW DOES THIS COMPARE TO SIMPLE DETOX AS EXPLAINED ABOVE?

Chelation is essentially all the same as it means to remove heavy metals from the body. The big difference is using harsh chemicals, which is very hard on the kidneys because it depletes all your good and bad minerals. Chelation is the ionic potential of specific minerals that creates natural cellular transportation in and out of the cell. When done at a slower rate, it's easy on the kidneys because it puts less demand on them. When you use seaweed and seawater, or ConcenTrace, it is more balanced with nature, so it's much less harmful on your kidneys. This is another good reason why I do the daily Detox Nutrient Mix.

CAN YOU TELL ME ABOUT FREE RADICALS WITH REGARD TO CELLS?

Free radicals are oxidizing agents that get inside the cell and change the mitochondrial function. The latest name for them is mitochondrial toxic epigenetic chemicals. The cells now become a cancerous cell or a pathogenic disease cell due to these radical chemicals' interference with the DNA and RNA communications, which will change the cells' function. And it's all coming from chemicals. There are over two hundred thousand chemicals the FDA and EPA have authorized to be used in our society today, plus the American Medical Association (AMA)-recommended drugs for diseases and illnesses. Then add processed foods and denaturing our foods by using a microwave to cook—both will lead to much less nutritional value. In our foods today, you get too much of one thing and not enough of another, and the outcome is, you're not healthy. As my pathology professor would say in medical school, "Either you adapt, or you die." Healthy Dad laughed and said, "Yes, you are getting it."

THERE IS *NO THINKING* OR WORRIES WITH WHOLE ORGANIC FOODS!

The most important thing to know about eating is to have the most nutritious food you can obtain. This will always be a diet based on organic whole grains and vegetables with some beans and legumes, and then you can add animal foods for flavoring in small amounts. Use condiments sparingly. Only use quality oils like virgin olive oil for salads and on vegetables. Use coconut oil for cooking. Sea salt is important as it has minerals that are important and essential to the body. It is best to cook it into the foods so you can taste the amount of sodium you are getting. Don't be afraid of salt, but only use sea salt in small or reasonable amounts.

Have some good bacteria regularly, even daily. This can be probiotics or fermented and cultured foods. This is the most important factor in digestion and your immune system.

WHAT IS THE DIFFERENCE BETWEEN ORGANIC AND NON-ORGANIC?

The label "organic" means it has been certified that no chemicals were used in the process of growing the crop from start to finish. It also means the crop was not from genetically modified seeds (GMO) that were made in a lab and altered to tolerate Roundup, which is used to kill weeds.

THE NUMBER ONE THING I HEAR FROM MY PATIENTS IS, ORGANIC COSTS TOO MUCH. WHAT WOULD YOU SAY TO THAT?

Can you put a price on your health? If you take the total cost of organic food over time, it will save you so much more money in the long run as compared to getting sick. The number one cost or expense when you retire is medical, and for those who do not have health insurance, it is even more costly. I feel the reason that someone has to work is to first put food on the table, but second, it is to have health insurance in case something goes wrong especially here in the United States.

Reflecting on what Healthy Dad said, maybe this is why I used the subtitle "What good is your wealth if you don't have your health?" I see so many of my patients, who, when they reach their retirement years, are now a slave to the ailment they have. They are on fifteen or more medications, they have to use a cane or walker to get around, or they're bound to a wheelchair or walker being attached to an oxygen tank. Just like my Sick Dad was when he retired to his recliner.

My Healthy Dad said, "I want to know what is in my food just like I want to know what is in my water." When you go with organic foods, it is better for you to eat foods that do not contain chemicals! One of the greatest tragedies is the poor quality of the food we consume. It's the main reason for disease.

HEALTHY DAD ASKED ME A QUESTION

Can you tell me where you have seen a case in your experience, working with the information I taught you, that if a person had followed what you are doing today, they would have not lost valuable time and money due to health?

Yes! I'm an example. My own personal experience where I lived on macaroni and cheese in college; root beer floats and Costco muffins in medical school; pizza and hot dogs in my residency; and all because it was so inexpensive. I was just trying to survive so one day I could thrive.

HEALTHY DAD THEN ASKED, "WHAT HAPPENED BY EATING THIS WAY? IT SOUNDS CHEAP AND CONVENIENT, BUT WHAT RESULTED?"

Well, my first episode occurred when I passed a kidney stone while in medical school, which led me to many tests, and then fighting for my life after having a reaction to the contrast dye study. I feel all of this was due to the way I was eating. Healthy Dad agreed that I was correct in my assessment.

WHAT PROTEINS DO YOU TAKE IN THE MORNING?

Proteins are units that the body can use to build more cells, but it does not only have to be in the morning. You want to consume proteins to rebuild and to heal. Here are some good ones: spirulina and eggs. When you eat protein for fuel, it will have to be broken down to be turned into fuel. Protein is made of carbon, hydrogen, oxygen, and nitrogen. Carbohydrates and fats are used for energy and are only made of carbon, hydrogen, and oxygen without the nitrogen.

In order for protein to be used for fuel, the nitrogen needs to be eliminated from the others in a process called ketosis. This floods the kidneys with too much nitrogen, and it is acidic. The kidney now has a problem mainly due to the lack of potassium used to eliminate it, which is one of the biggest problems that affects the heart and even results in kidney stones. In addition, it is inefficient as it takes energy to break the protein down to free the nitrogen, resulting in less energy you need to do the work that day.

HOW MANY HOURS SHOULD I WAIT TO GO TO BED AFTER EATING?

The liver/gallbladder works from about eleven o'clock in the evening to three o'clock in the morning—two hours for the gallbaldder and then two hours in the liver cycle as we learned in Chapter 4. The liver is like a chemical plant that processes all your blood chemicals so they are harmonious to the body tissues. During this four-hour period, the wood element needs to restore the purity of the blood. Eating will cause the liver to work on the food and not clean the blood as efficiently. This is why it is ideal not to eat three to four hours before going to bed.

Eating late at night or eating too large of an oily meal in the evening means your food may not get digested well before you go to bed. This will cause pressure in the blood flow through the liver, as well as too much blood going to the small intestine and therefore pooling the blood, which makes the heart have to beat harder to supply blood to the rest of the body. Both of these situations will elevate your blood pressure and disturb your sleep, as the heart will be working too hard to get deep rest. In oriental medicine, this is called disturbing the shen. You will notice this occurs about midnight to two o'clock in the morning, which is the liver peak time.

My response, "No wonder my body gave out in medical school! Doing all-nighters, staying up late, and eating at all hours of the night was doing more harm than good."

Continuing the discussion, my Healthy Dad went on to say, "Eating lighter or eating less at dinnertime will help you sleep better. Your liver restores you and sets everything back to the alkalinity, which purifies the cells. It is the way the body naturally heals itself and you can reset your body for the next day. Your liver restores that energy so it can meter out the glycogen from your liver. By having more whole grains in the morning, you will have a four-hour digestion time so that glucose will give you four hours of stable blood sugar. It protects your inheritance chi by effectively working on the nutrient chi, and a good night's sleep restores the prana chi. This balances all your three chi so they function on a sustainable level to give you a long healthy life."

WHAT ARE THE PRIMARY FACTORS OF HEALTH?

1. Lifestyle—What you do every day will affect your health. You can't remedy lifestyle means you cannot take a remedy and overcome a bad lifestyle!
2. Physical

3. Biological
4. Psychological
5. Energetic
6. Spirit
7. Purpose

This book mainly touches on the biological, which is the foundation for life.

IMPORTANT HEALTHY FACTORS TO HAVE AND DO

Here is a list of important factors to consider, some of which I have already mentioned. Items 1–8 have been discussed already; 9–10 are new subject matters but really are just common sense. This may be an area where you can start to develop your own questions.

1. **Quality of Water:** RO filtration = Know what is not in your water! I can add what I want in the water. What is reverse osmosis?
   A. According to the Atlantic Filter Corporation, reverse osmosis filters have an extremely tiny pore size—only 0.0001 microns. Therefore, reverse osmosis removes all organic molecules, viruses, most minerals, and monovalent ions. The end result is pure, desalinated water.
2. **Quality of Air Intake:** Deep breathing, ionic air from waterfalls, showers, plants, and air purifiers.
3. **Quality of Food:** Omega-3 HDL fats, proteins, carbohydrates, fruits, and vegetables for roughage.
4. **Quality of Minerals:** Sea and mineral salts, seawater, seaweed, and seafood, ConcenTrace liquid minerals.
5. **Good Bacteria:** Fermented foods and probiotics, such as yogurt, kefir, sauerkraut, and pickles.

6. **Food Preparation**: Yin-yang, hot vs. cold, cooked vs. raw; what your needs are to digest food. Don't forget chewing!
7. **Pace of Life**: Sleep, rest, exercise, and circadian rhythm; avoid blue light after dark.
8. **Attitude and Thoughts**: Objective vs. subjective, common sense, contemplation, prayer, and meditation.
9. **Exercise and Movement**: Structural freedom; stretching and manipulation; deep muscle therapy; quadrilateral motion like walking, swimming, and crawling; core tonin;, natural movement like gardening or house cleaning; tai chi; yoga; deep breathing; and calm or controlled rhythmic breathing.
10. **Natural Elements**: Being in nature. Sunlight, fresh air, grounding, touching the ground without insulation like rubber-soled shoes, being in water, and tree hugging (yes, it is okay to hug a tree even though it does not hug you back).

IMPORTANT HEALTHY FACTORS NOT TO HAVE OR DO

Items 1–6 and 9 have been discussed in previous chapters of the book. I added 7 and 8 to the list for you to research for yourself why I placed them here in the NOT to have or do section. I am only trying to get you to develop your own questions in your pursuits to a healthy lifestyle.

1. **Processed Foods**: Refined flour, vegetable oils, fried and fast food, snacks, and table salt.
2. **Sugars and Sweets**: Sugar, sweet fruits, syrups, white flour, potatoes, and artificial sweeteners.
3. **Fats and Oils**: Omega-6 LDL and omega-9 trans fats; vegetable oils, especially heated; and grain-fed hoofed animals like beef, lamb, buffalo, deer, and elk.
4. **Food and Water Chemicals**: Fluoride, chlorine, PVCs from

plastics, preservatives, additives, natural flavorings, and MSG.

5. **Chemicals:** Pharmaceutical drugs and endocrine disrupters, hormones, steroids, antibiotics, and glyphosate (Roundup). Vitamins are chemicals.

6. **Air Pollution:** Geo-engineering or chemtrails, ozone, indoor chemicals, cleaning products, textiles, and paint.

7. **Electrical and Magnetic Fields (EMFs) and Radio Frequencies (RFs):** Microwave devices like remote and cell phones, cell towers, Wi-Fi, Bluetooth devices, smart meters, 2G, 3G, 4G, and 5G, HAARP, house electrical wiring and high-voltage transmission wires, computers, electrical appliances, and tools.

8. **Vaccinations:** Chemicals, viruses, bacteria, and preservatives.

9. **Bad Attitudes, Negative Emotions, Thoughts, or Beliefs, Stress and Tension:** Thinking, worry, fear, apprehension, competition, trying to, overdoing mental or physical activity.

WHAT ARE THE BASIC NUTRITIONAL CONCEPTS OF QUALITY, PREPARATION, AND QUANTITY?

The following is listed in the order of importance:

- **Quality:** Organic grown with no chemicals or additives and especially avoid all genetically modified organisms (GMO) and genetically modified food (GMF). Organically grown food will increase the nutrient content by three to four times.

- **Food Preparation:** Ferment as many foods as you can to increase digestion and nutritional value. Cooked food is easier to digest. Cook meats and chicken in water and use the broth for stew. Raw food is weakening and cooling as well as harder to digest because it's harder to get the nutrition out of the plant.

- **Quantity**: Eat what you are hungry for. Higher nutritional food is more filling as you will not crave more. Know that if your food is low in nutritional value, you will want more food to fulfill the body's needs.

CONCLUSION

Quality means REAL food, PURE water, and CLEAN air! When you start to take shortcuts in life, life will find a way to cut you short. It is always important to know what is in your food and water. Treat your body with the utmost respect by eating and drinking the best quality food and water, and your life will be more enjoyable and pleasurable than what you can comprehend at this present moment. It is called health preservation instincts. When you make your decisions from your inner knowing and override your emotions, you will get healthier every day.

Do you know what was in your food and water today? How is your breathing? Do you breathe with your chest or your abdomen?

CHAPTER 7

Chemistry Is an Assault on Biology

———

Did Thomas Edison have a glass ball to the future when he said, **"The doctor of the future will give no medicine but will interest his patient in the care of the human frame, in diet, and in the cause and prevention of disease"?**

I find it amazing that the man who invented the light bulb also had the insight to pure and true nutrition. Here are a few scenarios to think about. We go to the gym for a workout, then we stop off at our favorite restaurant and eat to survive and socialize, never thinking twice about eating to thrive. We go to our doctor, whether naturopathic or modern medicine, and we get a pill to help us with our present illnesses to maintain our current lifestyle. We travel and we snack on things not knowing what we are eating.

This chapter will expose what is really attacking our human body with what we are eating. It will help you understand some very basic principles and misperceptions. This is the chapter with the information on which I spend most of my time with my patients when discussing nutritional concepts.

WHAT DO YOU MEAN BY CHEMISTRY IS AN ASSAULT ON BIOLOGY?

We have entered into a time where the prevailing thought is that chemistry and mathematics will fix everything. Here is a pill to fix your cold; here is a shot to protect you from the flu. When you add chemicals to your food to make "processed foods," biology does not have the ability to adapt. This causes an imbalance that alters the natural state of life (biology). Over time, this imbalance accumulates to create a dying organism. Just having the right lab numbers on a blood test does not ensure that you are a healthy person. In a good basic diet, if you have good bacteria and make sure the food is going to be digestible, then you're going to be healthy. If you put chemicals in it, you're **not** going to be healthy.

What does chemistry do? It kills your bacteria. What happens when your bacteria are destroyed? It makes it so you cannot digest any foods. And what does that do? It makes you sick. Biological life will be able to continue if left to the simple laws of nature. The less you do to your food chain, the more likely you will have a simple form of health, which results in less intervention to rebalance your health. If you mess with Mother Nature, she will send you to your room—*the hospital room!*

CAN YOU TELL ME MORE ABOUT GENETICALLY MODIFIED ORGANISMS?

One of the worst health problems we face at this present time in 2021 is the genetically modified organism (GMO) and glyphosate (Roundup). I have to put those two together because they are really one. Why? Because they can't live without each other. To keep it short, the side effects of glyphosate and GMOs are cancer, irritable bowel syndrome (IBS), digestive and immune problems, reproductive problems, liver damage, and emotional problems. You will start to see the third generation from your parents, which will be those born in 2030 and after, becoming more sterile. They will have more difficulty having children.

In 1973, genetic engineering was developed. In 1982, the FDA approved the first consumer product "human insulin" for treatment of diabetes. In 1994, the first GMO product was approved for sale for human consumption. In the 1990s, there was a mass flood of GMO products that became available to the consumer, such as soybeans, cotton, corn, papayas, tomatoes, potatoes, and canola. In 2003, the World Health Organization (WHO) allowed GMO internationally, and in 2015, the FDA allowed GMO in animal products, such as genetically engineered salmon.

Consumers rejecting GMO products is the only way we can stop the GMOs and Roundup. Furthering the discussion on GMO, my Healthy Dad went on to say, "I am going to stress, I am not as concerned with the GMOs as I am with the Roundup. The amount of GMO in your body you can eliminate better than you can Roundup. Roundup is patented as an antimicrobial, which kills the good microbe in the soil and in your intestines, which stops microbes from being able to change the minerals (especially iron, zinc, and magnesium) into a form the plants can absorb. So GMO plants have less nutrition, especially these minerals—iron, zinc, and magnesium, which are major nutrients the body needs. GMO plants have been genetically modified to be able to grow to full size in soil with less minerals. They look big, but they're like hollow balloons with not much nutrition; their weight is good, so it is all about the money. If your body doesn't have a good immune system and a good digestive system, then you're in trouble."

Let me make reference to it once again. Make sure you understand microbes digest and break down organic minerals in the soil and make it available for the plants to have organic compounds. This allows your body to have nutrients in their purest form. Healthy Dad wanted me to understand this often-confusing principle. GMO is designed to grow big without the need for those minerals because Roundup kills the microbes in the soil. Now you don't get enough minerals in that food. When you interfere with the microbes in the soil, you don't get these minerals. Those minerals are deficient in grains and beans that are GMOs because they have used Roundup on the soil to kill weeds that are not Roundup tolerant. These GMO foods will have much less nutritional value than what a normal or organic plant will have.

The other thing I will point out is Roundup is water-soluble, which means not only is it in the ground soil, but it is also in our air and in our water. It can go everywhere. Also, Roundup is used as a defoliant on wheat within ten days of harvesting to eliminate the weeds. It is on the grain and it's the major reason people have trouble with their digestive system. The concentration of Roundup on the grain is in a more active state and higher than when it is sprayed on the crop while they are growing.

Reflecting on what my Healthy Dad just said, I reflected on my Sick Dad's farm. The times we had a discussion he would tell me about other farmers who were using Roundup around his land, and over time, their crop yields had diminished. I could only assume that the soil was so depleted by the contamination by the Roundup that even the GMO seeds would not grow well. The other thing he pointed out was that the edges of his land were affected by the other farmers. If the other farmers would spray on a windy day, the Roundup would go over to the edges of his farmland. My Sick Dad was against using harsh chemicals in his crops because of his observation and knowledge of the soil in the area he farmed.

The bottom line was about the mighty dollar: more yield, more weight, more money in the farmer's pocketbook but more money in the pocketbooks of the pesticide and herbicide companies that sold to the farmers, too.

I would often hear the saying from my Sick Dad, "There is one occupation that God cursed from day one. Can you guess it? Yes, the farmers." Think about it: Adam and Eve were kicked out of the Garden and had to farm the land on their own. Now they faced weeds, drought, and insects, the land was cursed or punished, however you want to look at it. They did not have the luxury of having fruits and vegetables so readily in abundance in the garden where they once lived.

Healthy Dad went on to say the nutritional value is lacking in GMO products because Roundup makes those nutrients unavailable for the plant. The makers of Roundup designed a plant that can grow big without those nutrients. That means you don't get the good nutritional value from eating your foods. That's why people eat more because the food doesn't have enough nutrition and they crave more nutrition, so they eat more volume, then they gain weight because they are getting what we call hollow calories. What does that lead to? Diabetes, obesity, and heart disease!

Organic farms have microbes in the soils because there are no chemicals to kill them. These microbes and fungi create structures in the earth that cause the breaking down of the nutrients for plants. The fungus creates the structure of carbons that hold nutrients. The microbes create a somatic action that causes those vitamins and micronutrients to be held in the carbon structures of the fungus. When this happens, the plant matter turns into an available substance that the plant can grow on with its biological function. These plants will have the nutrients available for humans if they don't have chemicals applied to them that destroy this biological function.

CAN YOU TELL ME MORE AS TO HOW THE CHEMICAL ACTUALLY WORKS?

Most chemicals, pesticides, herbicides, and fungicides will injure the microbes in the soil. Most pesticides are hormones that interfere with the reproductive cycle of the bugs, and these hormones will affect humans. The final result is these chemicals causing a problem in your biology and destroying your bacteria. Then you don't get the nutrients out of the food you need, and you become sicker. There are over 200,000 chemicals authorized that are affecting our soils where our foods come from, with Roundup being the worst one yet. If you ignore the labels and let's say I just ate some yogurt thinking I am getting something good in my system, I am actually harming my body instead. If you don't eat yogurt that is from a grass-fed cow, in essence, you are getting hormones and Roundup because that cow had been fed grains that were GMO and sprayed with Roundup. This holds true for everything, including some fruits and vegetables. Now do you see why I say at least I want to know what is **NOT** in my food and water? I am trusting that at least the organic foods will give me some assurance that they are better than the regular things that are in the market. If you grow your own garden, you know what you're getting because you know what you're putting on it.

CAN YOU TELL ME WHAT TO AVOID AND WHAT TO BE AWARE OF WHEN I AM BUYING FOOD?

- Avoid soybeans, corn, canola, cottonseed, sugar beet products, and especially corn syrup or high-fructose corn syrup as 90 percent of these food products are GMO and have been sprayed with Roundup.
- Avoid animal products that are fed with GMO feed, hormones, and antibiotics: beef, pork, veal, sheep, chicken, turkey, eggs, lamb, or buffalo. All commercial feedlots use GMO feed products as well as hormones and antibiotics unless stated on the packaging.
- Avoid farm-raised fish: salmon, tilapia, and whitefish, because they have all been fed GMO products, and antibiotics. Salmon even has coloring agents added to make it red.
- Avoid nonorganic potatoes, alfalfa, Hawaiian papaya, crooked necked squash, zucchini, most sweet corn, and popcorn because they will be GMO and sprayed with Roundup.

It is best to look for Certified Natural (available in the northeast), then organic food locally grown (especially in-season foods), and animal foods that are humanely raised with space and no hormones or GMO feeds. Look for organic wheat, as regular whole wheat is defoliated with Roundup, and it is worse than even GMO products, as the glyphosate concentration is higher. This is why wheat is causing IBS; it's not the gluten. Italy does not use Roundup and people can eat the wheat there without problems, but not here in the United States.

WHY ARE SOME FOODS AFFECTED MORE THAN OTHERS WITH REGARD TO GMO AND ROUNDUP?

If you're a weak individual, you don't have good bacteria, and if you don't have good health, then you are vulnerable. Your immune system is already weak and now GMO and Roundup make it more problematic, which will cause you to end up getting allergies, cancer, diabetes, or chronic infections. You also may have brain chemistry problems such as Alzheimer's, autism, and ADHD.

WHAT ARE SOME EXTERNAL FACTORS AFFECTING OUR HEALTH?

Staying on the topic of chemicals, I was curious to know what else besides plants and animals affects our health when exposed to chemicals.

As mentioned before, I did not suffer from asthma until after I was vaccinated with the MMR at the age of four. When you find out how many problems have originated from Type 1 diabetes, it's in the immunizations. Yes! Because what is put in the vaccines causes the body to attack itself. We call it an autoimmune disease. Diabetes Type 1 is autoimmune; it's coming from the vaccines that are being given. The mercury, aluminum, and some fifty other things they are adding to the injectable are causing harm to the human body. This is the great debate and very controversial, so do your own homework. You will hear both sides pleading their cases, but know this: When someone gets injured from a pill from a pharmaceutical company, they can sue for damages; however, the vaccination companies are exempt. If any case goes to court, it is the taxpayers that end up paying the bill if the case settles because the plaintiff is actually suing the government and not the pharmaceutical company that developed the vaccine because the government passed a hidden protection clause in a spending bill for the manufacturers of the vaccines in 1986, and now the taxpayer via the government pays the settlements.

Vaccines have a dead virus in them, and these viruses don't trigger your immune system to recognize the pathogen. You don't become immune to that specific pathogen.

How does a person make themselves immune without vaccines? The answer is, "herd immunity." By being exposed to the pathogen and having a good immune system, you will develop lifelong antibodies to it.

Reflecting on what I have been told, it wasn't until I was at the age of four when I was first vaccinated with the MMR. It was right after this when I started with my asthma symptoms. I was not like the other kids. I wanted to run and be like them. Throughout my elementary and high school years, I would have to rely on my asthma inhaler so I could participate in sports. Was it the vaccination that triggered an attack on my own body? Why did my older brother go into a full-blown reaction when he received the smallpox vaccination and had to have the antiserum life-flighted in to save his life?

I am not against vaccinations if I know what is in them and the vaccine has been proven truthful in a double-blind study by credible third-party scientists with the specific vaccine.

When my little girl at a very young age was stung by a bark scorpion, I was hesitant to have her get the antiserum because I had heard of a small boy who was also stung by the same type of scorpion died from the complication of the injection just months before she was stung. Watching my daughter and listening to the ER doctor, I made the choice to give my daughter the antiserum (a specific injectable for a specific condition) when the doctor was running out of choices. She survived this scare, and I am very thankful for the ER doctor who was there at the time of my daughter's incident.

There will be many questions that linger in my mind raised by the many books and articles that have been published pertaining to vaccinations. One question I have is why is it that a child will have at least twenty to thirty to even up to seventy vaccinations by the time they are eight years old? There are those out there who have devoted their entire life to taking on the vaccination companies, and I will leave it to you, the reader, to research for yourself both sides of the debate and then formulate your own opinion on the matter.

IS IT POSSIBLE TO GET RID OF THESE TOXINS IN YOUR BODY?

Yes, you can. I have discussed with you how to eliminate with nutrition, which is based on the nutrient detox mix and the immune diet. These are effective in taking out heavy toxins by a natural chelation process. I once knew a man whose legs were very dark gray because he was a welder for more than twenty-five years (1950–77). He would breathe in all these heavy toxic metals at work on a daily basis. After applying the heavy metal diet, his legs had almost returned to a normal color in six months just by changing what he was eating. My Healthy Dad said he was one of the worst heavy metal individuals that he has ever worked with. This nutritional approach of using the heavy metal diet naturally chelates (removes) the heavy metals out of the body.

Note to the reader: The heavy metal diet is not mentioned in this book as it is very specific to the individual. It is one of over forty diets that I have seen for various specific ailments. Chapters 9–11 will expose you to the immune diet, the diabetic diet, and the whole life diet. These are the most common ones I use in my practice.

If you would like more information on this specific diet that is not mentioned in detail in this book, you may refer to my website www.liveitlifestyles.com for a full description.

CAN I JUST TAKE SUPPLEMENTS TO STAY HEALTHY?

You cannot remedy a lifestyle! You cannot rely on a pill to fix your problem. The world as we know it has changed. We have entered into this Aquarian age, and it will be with us for another 2,000 years. We just came out of the Piscean age that was around for 2,000 years. The Aquarian age is personal responsibility, meaning you are going to have to take responsibility for yourself. Start asking more questions and take an active role in your life. It is not about finding the holy grail or taking this magical pill or supplement that will somehow fix all your health problems. It now depends on adopting a lifestyle change. This is a major commitment on your part, so you will have to make your health a priority.

You've got to eat right! You can't get away with taking a supplement and not changing your lifestyle.

You have to participate! You cannot remedy a lifestyle which means, "Your holy grail is your holy grill!" Quit relying on someone else and take an active role in your life. This all sounds good, but you will need good role models along the way who can lead you in the right direction.

Healthy Dad said when you ask the questions, take responsibility for yourself, do the discipline, eat right, get some sleep, add the right fluids, think right, have a purpose in life, do some exercise and keep your body moving (I mean movement in life. Do what it takes to keep moving; quadrilateral stretching is a great place to start), you will start to see your transformation into a healthy lifestyle. It will be your responsibility to want it and to start the process, but the rewards are priceless!

Just know you can't take a drug, get surgery, or take a healthy pill and expect to keep the same lifestyle you've always had. Making the choice today is the first step.

WHAT IS THE BUCKET THEORY?

Healthy Dad would always talk about the bucket theory, which developed into wanting to know about cleaning the bucket. I asked my Healthy Dad what is the meaning of cleaning the bucket?

The bucket theory is this: Your body is like a bucket of muddy water. How do you get the water clear in the bucket? You stick a hose in the bucket, turn the water on, and wait until you get clear water.

How long does it take for the bucket to get clean? "Well, it depends on how much water is coming in and how muddy the water is in the bucket."

Some buckets are large, and some buckets are small. Some buckets have more clean water coming in while others just have a trickle. It's all just a matter of time until the bucket becomes clean. So when you work with people, they will all have a different bucket, and they will all have water coming in. It is your challenge to get them to ask the questions so their hose with water coming in is no longer just a trickle.

There are parameters of your situation that will determine when you feel good, which means your bucket is clear, and when you don't feel good, which is when your bucket is not clean. Keep the clear water coming in, and eventually, you can get rid of the toxic mud. Now we have things that will accelerate the process. Good quality minerals, good quality food, and then a few other tricks get your body working, such as elimination and good rest. The clear water in your bucket is your plasma and your blood. The bucket is your body. So when you get your body clear, you get your cells clean. Then everything is in harmony, so health is a given. It's the law of nature.

EXACTLY HOW DO CELLS IN THE BODY WORK?

Healthy Dad explained, "It is called mitochondrial epigenetics."

I thought maybe he was just making up words. I said, "Epigenetic what? They never used that terminology in medical school when I was there." Mitochondrial epigenetics is a fancy new word meaning, "the chemicals that affect the cell function." It's the function of the cell. These are chemicals in the cell that affect how it will perform its function. If you have good epigenetic chemicals, you have good cellular function. They call this mitochondrial epigenetics. The mitochondria are the engines in the cells that utilize nutrients. If you have bad chemicals going into the cell, the mitochondria don't have a good function.

Here is an example. Imagine building your house out of ice in Arizona. How long is that going to last until ice turns into water? Not very long because it's always warm there. The mitochondria are everything in the house, and the epigenetic is the ice or everything outside. They are the chemicals that affect the mitochondrial function. Every cell is different from one another in function and purpose. Within each cell, the mitochondria know the work or function they are supposed to do. The mitochondria will not function well because of the bad chemicals, and they may do something completely different than the cell is programmed to do for the whole body. What happens is the house in which the mitochondria live is now in disarray, and the house is no longer functioning as a unit. There will be some houses that have completely collapsed, while others will take on the new strangers and their energy and start to act like them and thus become a toxic environment and eventually die.

The biology in your cells all work for one reason; they have the same goal. They all do different jobs, but they all work for the housekeeping function. They all have a purpose for the total: "the organism." They're all doing something to make the house work in a normal manner.

Every cell in your entire body has a mitochondrial cell. They are the workers within the cell, and those workers do what they are told to do when there is complete harmony. When the bucket is clear and clean, the mitochondria work is epigenetics, the cellular nutritional needs for the cell function are in balance. When there are no bad chemicals introduced into the cell, it now produces what the genetic information is designed to do and goes to work for the whole body.

Taking this information and now doing my own research on the subject, I wanted to know some of the chemicals that were affecting my body. This led me to one chemical that I see affecting so many people in my clinic.

One day, I had a patient who came into my office with unexplained pain. The first thing she said to me was, "You are now the sixth or seventh doctor I've been to for this constant pain in my legs and feet. What can you do for me?"

Taking a deep breath, I started to ask her my questions to help me formulate a workable solution. I asked her the typical pain questions such as: Is the pain worse at night or during the day? Describe the pain to me. Is it constant or sporadic? Is there anything that may bring it on, such as exercise or just plain walking? Describe the pain to me. Is it sharp or is it burning? After I got done with my questions, I then went into the examination.

This patient presented differently from others. Most of the time, I can figure out in a very quick manner if there is a nerve that is irritated or if it is coming from more of a systemic presentation, such as neuropathy, or if it was something that was out of alignment, such as an ankle, knee, or midfoot. When nothing was adding up, a thought came to me. Could this be that simple? Is she being poisoned by the food she is eating?

I then asked her a question: "Do you eat or drink anything with the term 'diet' in it, such as diet soda?"

She then turned to me and said, "Yes, I drink two six-packs of Diet Pepsi a day."

I told her to go home and get rid of all the remaining diet soda that she had. I told her not to drink anything with an ingredient called aspartame, NutraSweet, or Splenda. She agreed, and then I scheduled her to come back in two weeks.

When she showed up to my clinic, I walked into the room and had to do a double take because she did not appear to be in distress or in pain. I asked her how she was feeling, and she said, "I have no pain at all. The pain is gone!" I have found that artificial sugars will exacerbate systemic conditions such as fibromyalgia. In her case, I would have to go back to see if she had an underlying systemic condition, but what I can tell you is, once she stopped the artificial sugars, the pain stopped.

WHAT ARE JUNK OILS?

Junk oils are ones that have been extracted by toxic solvents; the high pressure makes them more rancid. For instance, junk oils include canola oil and all the cooking oils that people use and products like soy, corn, and cottonseed. These are your main oils that are GMO. They are very inexpensive. When you use these oils, you will have wood meridian problems, which is liver problems, because you're not going to be able to digest those fats well. They will cause congestion in the liver and then they'll get stuck in your body in the fat cells that are close to your organs. Eventually, this will result in potential cancers. The other problem with junk oils is, they are acidic. This will cause avascular inflammation, just as junk sugars will.

HOW DO JUNK OILS AFFECT THE LIVER?

Over the course of time, the inability to utilize the oils will result in the body slowing down and the liver energy dropping, so you end up feeling sluggish. If the blood cannot get through the liver due to the congestion from junk oils, a person will eventually lose ambition and have less energy. Over time, junk oil congestion will also create Alzheimer's and circulation problems such as strokes. It creates an inability for the body to function well emotionally.

Because the liver is rational behavior, a bad liver is irrational.

The liver is the seat of emotional anger and aggression. A perfect example as mentioned before in the previous chapter is the difference between first degree and second degree murder. First degree is the imbalance of the heart, something that was thought out, premeditated, and second degree murder is the imbalance of the liver, a spontaneous explosion, a reaction! If you commit first degree murder (heart) you are sentenced for life or receive the death sentence, whereas if you commit second degree murder (liver), it is a term sentence or shorter period of time.

In summary, junk oils on this liver will cause a fatty liver, a fatty heart, and fatty intestines and a place where chemicals are stored. This physical result includes cancers, heart conditions, and bad immune systems. The liver is on the wood meridian and so you will see outbursts, anger, impatience, frustrations, and aggression adding to but not completely caused by the tension. This is the result of ingesting bad oils that congest the liver. This is a classic example of the five element principle and emotional behavior.

WHAT IS THE DIFFERENCE BETWEEN A WHITE PIMPLE AND A RED PIMPLE?

White pimples are too yin, too much white flour, too much dairy that is not being digested. That is the mucus coming through the skin. This is a lung/large intestine involvement. People with white pimples are not digesting their proteins.

When you have a red pimple, it is their liver/gallbladder. These are from not digesting your fats. You are eating too much heated oils, french fries, and potato chips. If you have a sensitive liver, then you will have more red pimples.

WHAT ARE THE DHA (DOCOSAHEXAENOIC ACID), EPA (EICOSAPENTAENOIC ACID), AND ALA (ALPHA-LINOLENIC ACID)?

These are all essential omega-3 fatty acids; DHA and EPA are from animal fats, and ALA are from plants. Vegetable oils don't have any DHA or EPA. Omega-3 is like detergent whereas the omega-6 and omega-9 fatty acids are like grease. Omega-6 and omega-9 don't break down without omega-3 fatty acids. These types of fats don't have the ability to metabolize themselves, and they turn into glycogen and triglycerides. Triglycerides get stored in the fat cells and they're like a magnet for chemicals. In addition, all those chemicals are in an oxidized state. The more air, heat, rancidness, and volatility results in health problems including diabetes, heart disease, and cancers. One way you can tell if you're eating bad fats is by the red and white pimples. Trans fats will give you red pimples, and white pimples come from indigestible proteins. There are many chemicals we unknowingly put into our bodies every day.

CONCLUSION

By understanding more and asking more questions, we become better educated.

Medical school never had a single course in nutrition and yet it produces outstanding surgeons and physicians. If Thomas Edison could see what he said over one hundred years ago, even he would be amazed by his statement.

My questions to you are the following: What is in your bucket? Is it clear, or is it muddy? If you cook at home, what oils do you use? If you eat out a lot, have you ever stopped to think if what you are eating is nutritional?

In the next chapter, we will explore more of these chemicals and how to recognize them. We will see their effects, and we will learn to read the labels when we're in the grocery store. I will also show you what is in your food and some of the tricks used in the food industry.

CHAPTER 8

Read It before You Eat It!

———

Did you know that food companies will use ways to sell their products by packing more sugar into their product without you even knowing about it by just using words on the pacakge to make you think you're buying something healthy? Did you know that harmful ingredients take on new names in the products you're buying?

Eating is a necessity for a human to survive, but how many of us actually read the labels of what we eat? There has never been a greater need for this than this time right now. In taking on personal responsibility, it is up to us to ask the questions and know what is in our foods, especially when we eat out.

DO WE ACTUALLY KNOW WHAT IS IN OUR FOOD?

In working with patients, I am amazed that even the healthiest people do not read food labels for what they eat. It has been a practice of mine to read the labels before buying anything. I will even ask the organic restaurants if they use any junk oils or ingredients other than what they advertised. Some of the questions I will ask are as follows: Is the beef grass-fed? Are the buns organic whole grain? Is the salmon farmed or wild caught? What is in the salad dressings? My Sick Dad never asked what was in the food he ate. I never once saw him look at a label on the ice-cream box, candy bar wrapper, or the soda drink.

Recently, I had a patient who came into my office who suffered from gout. It had been going on for several weeks. He informed me that he did not eat red meat, nor did he drink any alcohol. When I asked him if he was eating anything with corn syrup or high-fructose corn syrup, the patient said, "I don't eat any of that." I asked if he'd had a bowl of ice cream the previous night. When he said he did, I told him to go back home and read every package on every food item he was eating and then let me know at the next appointment.

When the patient came back, he was very happy. He was not suffering from pain because of the treatment I rendered on the initial visit. He was amazed at how many food items contained corn syrup.

HOW MANY OF US READ THE FOOD LABELS OF WHAT WE BUY?

This is a question for you. When you went to the grocery store or your local market on the corner, did you just grab the items and go, or did you take the time to really read what you were about to purchase? Life today is so convenient. Think about it: everything is prepared for us. We do very little food preparation or cooking anymore. All we have to do is take the item out of the bag, throw it in a microwave, and then eat it.

DO WE ASK WHAT IS IN THE FOOD WE ORDER AT RESTAURANTS WHEN WE EAT OUT?

Here in America, we are so dependent on restaurants to prepare our meals for us. We grab our breakfast on the way to work. At lunch, it takes us longer to walk across the street than it does to have our lunch prepared for us after we order it. And yet we never ask what is in our food. Personally, I love eating out at restaurants, but I am very careful in choosing which ones I go to. I have gone out to eat with my Healthy Dad, but he uses each experience as a teaching opportunity. When we go out to eat, he will research which restaurants serve brown rice and organic foods. When we are at the restaurants, he will get a glass of bottled water or a tea that is organic. Eating out is more of a social thing and so most of our time is spent talking and discussing subjects during the actual dinner portion. We usually skip the dessert unless it is made of fine quality foods that only use organic ingredients. By the time we have chewed our food twenty times before swallowing during the main portion of the meal, we are usually too full to get dessert anyway.

NATURAL FLAVORING

The use of the word "natural" on food labels is something of a joke because it means so little. Natural really means it tastes like natural! Many highly processed foods can be called "natural." Unlike "organic," there isn't an official verification process companies have to go through before using the term.

Anna Roth, in an article titled "5 Things to Know About the 'Dark Act'" and published July 20, 2015, notes that "a *Consumer Report* survey found that nearly 60 percent of shoppers look for the 'natural' label on foods and more than 75 percent of them believe that the label has specific attributes like lack of artificial coloring, flavor, or GMOs." People think "natural" means that their food is safe, but there is actually no legal definition for natural. Anything can be "natural"!

WHAT ABOUT CORN SYRUP?

I asked my Healthy Dad about corn syrup. He said, "Corn syrup and high-fructose corn syrup and fructose sugar are all the same thing." Developed by a Japanese scientist, it was introduced to the United States during the Nixon administration because regular cane sugar was so expensive, and a cheaper sugar was needed at the time.

Found in soda, ice cream, bread, baby formula, and fast foods, it's one of the main single food ingredients that is causing childhood obesity and diabetes. Corn syrup is sold under the notion that it is safe and causes no harm since it is a simple sugar. However, the digestive process is not the way same as simple sugar is. When a sugar molecule gets into our body, it goes into our intestine and then into our liver for processing. When a corn syrup molecule hits the liver, the liver thinks it is a simple sugar molecule and so it proceeds through the Krebs cycle (energy conversion cycle) for processing. Upon delivery, however, the liver cannot break it down fully. When a molecule cannot be broken down into glycogen and then on to either energy or stored in a fat cell, it is turned it into uric acid as a waste product. Corn syrup will create a lot of uric acid in the body, which leads to gout, diabetes, and many other ailments.

WHAT IS THE DIFFERENCE BETWEEN GLUTEN-FREE AND NON-GMO?

GMO means genetically modified organism or food. Gluten is

the protein in wheat. Wheat, unless it's organic, is defoliated with Roundup/glyphosate even though wheat is non-GMO. It is not the gluten that is causing the irritable bowel and digestive problems but the nonorganic wheat we eat that has Roundup on it.

You may think you're helping your body by eating gluten-free, but unless what you eat is organic, you are still harming your gut by killing your good bacteria.

WHAT ARE SOME OF THE INVISIBLE GMO INGREDIENTS IN FOODS AND PACKAGED FOOD?

Craig Thursday, in an article titled "GMOs—Take Them Back to the Store," published in *Real Health Talk* on November 15, 2012, shares the following information: Most food products will have GMO and Roundup in them, unless all the ingredients are organic and labeled non-GMO. Here is a list of the most common GMO foods and the worst offenders: soy, corn, cotton oils, canola oils, sugar beets, and potatoes. And now many other foods are being developed.

These ingredients are full of Roundup and are GMOs: baking powder, caramel color, casein, cellulose, condensed milk, confectioner's sugar, corn flour, corn masa, cornmeal, corn oil, corn sugar, corn syrup, fructose, high-fructose corn syrup, cornstarch, cyclodextrin, cysteine, dextrin, dextrose, diacetyl, diglyceride, erythritol, Equal, food starch, glucose, glutamate, glutamic acid, glycerides, glycerin, glycerol, glycerol monooleate, hemicellulose, hydrolyzed starch, inverse syrup, inverted sugar, isoflavones, lactic acid, lecithin, leucine, lysine, maltitol, malt, malt syrup, malt extract, maltodextrin, maltose, mannitol, methylcellulose, milk powder, milo starch, modified food starch, modified starch, mono- and diglycerides, monosodium glutamate (MSG), NutraSweet, aspartame, amino-sweet oleic acid, phenylalanine, phytic acid, protein isolate, tamari, tofu, miso, tempeh, teriyaki marinade, texturized vegetable protein (TVP), hydrolyzed protein, autolyzed yeast threonine, tocopherols (vitamin E), triglyceride, whey, whey powder, vegetable fat, vegetable oil, vitamin B12, xanthan gum, and natural flavorings.

The next time you go to the grocery store, I want you to look at the label and ask yourself, "Does it say natural flavoring? Does it contain soy, corn, or beets that are genetically modified? Is it organic? Are there words I cannot pronounce?"

So just know anything you cannot pronounce or do not recognize contains GMO and/or Roundup. If you can't read it, don't eat it. Plain and simple!

WHAT OTHER ADDITIVES AND INGREDIENTS IN OUR FOOD ARE HARMFUL TO US?

Ever wonder what is really in the food at the grocery store? In the following descriptions are some of the more common food items we eat without even knowing the harm they are doing to us. This information comes from an article by Mike Adams, titled "What's Really in the Food? The A to Z of the Food Industry's Most Evil Ingredients," published on July 31, 2011.

Acrylamides—Toxic, cancer-causing chemicals that form when carbohydrates are exposed to high heat (baking, frying and grilling). They are present in everything from bread crusts to snack chips, and because they are not intentional ingredients, acrylamides do NOT have to be listed on labels.

Aspartame—A chemical sweetener that causes neurological disorders, seizures, blurred vision, and migraine headaches. Can be also be referred to as NutraSweet, Equal, Canderel, Amino-Sweet and E951. Hospitals will commonly give diabetics aspartame as a substitute for sugar.

BPA (Bisphenol-A)—A hormone-mimicking chemical found in nearly all food packaging plastics. Tiny trace amounts (just parts per billion!) are enough cause problems. BPA has been linked to cancer, infertility, hormone disruption, and male breast growth.

Casein—Milk proteins. Ironically, casein is widely used in "soy cheese", which is promoted as an alternative to dairy.

Food Colors—FD&C Red #40, also called Allura Red AC, has been shown to cause behavior disorders. Most artificial food colors are derived from petroleum and are contaminated with aluminum.

Genetically Modified Ingredients—Not currently listed on food labels, although federally-mandated GMO labels are scheduled to go into effect in 2022. The most common GMO crops are corn, soy, cotton, and sugar beets; GMO corn is so widespread that if you're not eating organic corn, it's impossible to avoid GMO corn. GMOs have been linked to severe infertility problems and may even cause the bacteria in your body to produce and release a pesticide in your own gut.

High Fructose Corn Syrup/HFCS/Corn Syrup—A highly processed liquid sugar extracted from corn with the chemical solvent glutaraldehyde and frequently contaminated with mercury. HFCS has been linked to obesity, diabetes, and mood disorders. It's hard to avoid, because it's used not just in candy and sweets, but in things you wouldn't expect, like spaghetti sauce or salad dressing.

Homogenized Milk—The fats in the milk are artificially modified so the fat molecules are smaller and stay in suspension in the liquid rather than separating. It makes milk look better on the shelf, but it's also blamed for promoting heart disease and may contribute to milk allergies. Raw milk is healthier.

Hydrochloride—A chemical form of vitamin B added to food products so that the daily value of vitamins per serving appears higher. These are synthetic vitamins, not natural (derived from plants or animals). Nutrionally, they are almost useless. In fact, they may actually be bad for you. Also watch out for synthetic forms of vitamin B12 (niacinamide and cyanocobalamin).

Hydrolyzed Vegetable Protein—A highly processed form of soy protein that's used as a taste enhancer.

Partially Hydrogenated Oils—Oils that are modified using a chemical catalyst to make them stable at room temperature; this process creates trans fatty acids, more commonly known as "trans fats." Trans fats are junk oils that are stable at room temperature, resulting in trans fatty acids that greatly increase the risk of blocked arteries.

Phosphoric Acid—The acid used in sodas to dissolve the carbon dioxide; it adds to the overall fizziness of the soda. But phosphoric also acid has other uses: masons use it to etch rocks and the military uses it to clean the rust off battleships. If it can etch a rock, it will definitely destroy your tooth enamel.

Propylene Glycol—A liquid used in to winterize RVs. When combined with artificial colors and corn syrup, it's used to make the fake blueberries you find in blueberry muffins, bagels, bread, popcorn, and fast foods.

Sodium—White salt, which has been processed and lacks trace minerals. Not to be confused with "dirty" sea salt or pink Himalayan salt, which are loaded with trace minerals such as selenium, chromium, and zinc. Sodium in the form of white salt is terrible for your health. Don't be fooled by salt labeled "sea salt" at the grocery story—since all salt came from the sea at some point, food companies can label any salt "sea salt," no matter how much it's processed.

Sodium Nitrite—A cancer-causing red coloring added to nearly all processed meat, such as bacon, lunch meat, pepperoni, and hot dogs.

Soy Protein—A "junk protein" commonly used in protein bars. Soy protein is made from GMO soybeans by processing them with hexane, an explosive chemical solvent.

Sucralose—An artificial sweetener, most commonly called Splenda. The sucralose molecule contains chlorine. Though it is promoted as a diet food, researchers have found that sucralose and other artificial sweeteners actually promote weight gain.

Sugar—The bleached by-product of cane processing. When sugar cane is processed, nearly all the vitamins and minerals end up in blackstrap molasses, leaving white sugar nutritionally deficient. Blackstrap molasses is actually the 'good' part of sugar cane juice. Sugar promotes diabetes, obesity, mood disorders, and nutritional deficiencies.

Textured Vegetable Protein—Usually made of soy protein, which is extracted from genetically modified soybeans and then processed using hexane. Widely used in vegetarian foods, such as "veggie burgers."

Yeast Extract—A hidden form of MSG that contains up to 14 percent free glutamate. Many so-called "natural" products use yeast extract so they can claim their products contain no MSG. Can be found in thousands of grocery store products, from soups to chips to fast food.

FOOD LABEL TRICKS OR HOW TO READ A LABEL

Food companies uses several tricks when writing labels to make foods seem healthier than they are. Watch out for these tricks when you're reading labels!

First Trick: According to Mike Adams, food companies use this trick to pack more sugar into their products without making sugar look like the main ingredient. Ingredient labels must list the most prominent ingredients first, and some consumers might hesitate to buy a box of cereal that listed sugar as the first ingredient. So, a food company will use three or four different forms of sugar so they can be listed separately, and therefore appear further down the label. For example, a cereal might list it's primary ingredients as "whole grain wheat, sugar, corn syrup, corn syrup solids..." The cereal seems healthy, because the first ingredient is "whole grain wheat." However, in reality, the cereal might contain over 50 percent sugars!

Second Trick: Another way food labels will be manipulated through a trick is name changing. If the name of an ingredient has been given a bad rap, then a new name will replace it, even though the chemical makeup is still identical. Aspartame is an ingredient that carries many other names, such as Amino-Sweet. Corn syrup is also another one. It is sometimes called fructose sugar or high-fructose corn syrup, making you think you're getting good sugar from fruit.

Third Trick: Enticing wordage, such as **enriched** corn meal, **vegetable** oil, **natural** flavor. These entice you to think the ingredients are good for you, but in reality, they are the opposite.

WHAT CAN YOU TELL ME ABOUT ANTIOXIDANTS?

Most of what you hear about antioxidants is good. But they only work if they come in a whole food form because synergistic nutrients found in whole foods are needed to activate them. They are not used as well by the body when taken in a pill. So eat fresh fruits and vegetables for the best source. Berries are the best, but all veggies have them. Dark greens and freshly juiced veggies are best, but even powdered spirulina, chlorella, blue-green algae, barley, alfalfa, or wheatgrass will work. Most teas have antioxidants; rooibos is the best, having five times more antioxidants than green tea. There is no need to buy expensive supplements to get these antioxidants, as dark greens and fresh fruits have them in forms that are more usable by the body.

HOW CAN I BUY HONEST FOOD?

- The most important thing to do is ask questions, such as, "What is in the food?" and "How is it grown?"
- Start your own garden on the porch or in the yard. There are more and more support groups out there that can give you great gardening advice.

- Shop at your local farmers' market. Most communities will have them; just ask around.
- Always look for the USDA label on foods that says "organic."
- Read it before you eat it! Before you even put any item in the grocery cart, read the label.
- Make your own meals at home using fresh and organic ingredients. When you buy those ready-to-be-made packages that you can throw in the microwave, just know they are full of chemicals in most cases.

WHAT CAN YOU TELL ME ABOUT FLUORIDE AND WHAT IT DOES TO US?

Fluoride is an industrial waste that is too toxic to dump in the water or land fields. Now they put it into our toothpaste, and we are told that it is good for our teeth. It calcifies the pineal gland, it slows down the ability to think, and it shuts down the intuitive faculty. You become prone to more programming. Everyone needs to understand fluoride and chlorine are poisons. In the United States, fluoride was added to most municipal water supplies and bottled waters and we have been told it is safe and healthy for us. This is one area of controversy in our health. Personally, I will take all possible measures to avoid fluoride. One of the main reasons is that fluoride calcifies the pineal gland or higher cognitive thinking, and in high dosages it can be linked to cancer. I feel it ranks up there for one of the toxins we most need to avoid.

WHAT CAN YOU TELL ME ABOUT THE PINEAL GLAND?

How does the pineal gland come into play? The pineal gland is the seventh chakra or the higher self. The pineal gland is how you connect to a higher consciousness or awareness.

IS THERE A TERM FOR WHEN THE PINEAL GLAND DOES NOT FUNCTION OR IS DAMAGED?

Yes, it is called calcification, and this is caused by the chemical fluoride. The pineal gland has a liquid in it, which gives the "inner knowing" more potential; thus, when the pineal gland starts to calcify, the ability to know oneself becomes more difficult. Everyone needs a purpose and true hope in life. When your pineal gland is working, you are more aware and can formulate questions to ask as you take this journey in life. What is important to understand is omega-3 oils, along with chemical-free balanced nutrition, will help to decalcify the pineal gland.

WHAT ABOUT SUPPLEMENTS? CAN'T I JUST TAKE A PILL AND BE ASSURED I AM GOING TO BE HEALTHY? WHAT CAN YOU TELL ME ABOUT SUPPLEMENTS?

Most supplements are too concentrated and/or chemically extracted, so they are toxic to the liver. These will not give you health in the long run. Your liver will actually need to process them for good health. At best, you will not generally benefit from them, and at worst, they will make you sicker. **Remember, *"Chemistry is an assault on biology."*** Anything that is man-made has a chemical trail attached to it whether it be the plastic digestible pill container or some additive that is used to keep the pills fresh.

WHAT CAN YOU TELL ME ABOUT VITAMINS?

Vitamins are important. However, just like with antioxidants, they are good when they comes from the true synergistic source of nature but not from a secondhand source (chemically processed). The body will decide that day what it needs and absorb it, and then what it does not need, it will let it pass through the digestive system to be eliminated even if it is good nutrition. Note: Mineral concentrates do have a value in the daily intake, as organic foods today may not have the nutritional value that foods did one hundred years ago.

As far as vitamins and herbs go, they are health supplements. They will only be helpful for a limited period of time medicinally and then they become nutritive and will no longer have the medicinal effect.

The vitamins you take on a daily basis are too concentrated and will give the liver and intestines trouble. The pH in your system will be off, so they will make it more difficult to grow good bacteria in your gut. The liver will have to work harder to process them and it is harder for the kidney to eliminate them. A classic example is when a high dose of vitamin C is taken; it actually kills the good bacteria in the stomach and small intestine and does more harm than good. Vitamins don't change the chemistry of the body that is off because of poor diet, so know if you haven't changed the cause, taking them is just wasting your money. They say Americans have the richest urine because they pee out everything they just spent on supplements.

Healthy Dad reminded me that "money is easy to make. Integrity is hard to keep." I've never sold supplements.

Healthy Dad ran a health food store from 1974 to 1976 and there were no pills allowed in the store. Heathy Dad said, "I've lived this way for about fifty years now. It's not magic; it's just cleaning the bucket! And then make sure the bucket doesn't get dirty again! And you'll be healthy!"

CONCLUSION

In my practice, I am amazed by the statement from my patients who say, "I eat healthily, so why do I have diabetes, gout, and fungal infections?" My standard answer is, "Read it before you eat it!" When I explain what to look for in their foods, they will come back to me and say, "I did not know how much corn syrup was in everything!" or "I am now reading everything before I put it in my shopping cart!" We must be more educated in what we eat. If we are putting trust in others to tell us what is in our foods, then we are missing a valuable principle. To take up this personal responsibility, we must take an active role in what we are eating.

One thing I often repeat to my patients is, "Read it before you eat it!" When you go to the grocery store, would you put on a blindfold and just pick things off the shelf and put them in your basket? You most likely wouldn't, but when you don't read the labels on the food you're buying, you're basically doing the same thing. How many of you actually look at the labels before buying?

There are three rules of nutrition, and they will always protect you from bad things.

1. Read it before you eat it!
2. If you cannot read it, don't eat it!
3. If it tastes good, spit it out! (I know you needed a good laugh after reading this chapter! It is said laughter is the best medicine!)

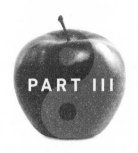

PART III

The Formats for the Immune Diet, the Diabetic Diet, and the Whole Life Diet

CHAPTER 9

What Good Is Your Wealth if You Don't Have Your Health?

Live-It Lifestyles for the Immune Diet and Reestablishing the Digestive Bacteria

---

INTRODUCTION

I have always said you cannot put a price on your health, but inevitably we do it every day. We are trained to look at the price of the food item we are buying and yet we never look at the ingredients.

I will share three diets in this book. These three diets are the ones most commonly needed by my patients; other diets for other specific problems can be found at www.liveitlifestyles.com. The first, covered in this chapter, is the immune diet, best for the yin person. Next is the diabetic diet, which is both yin and yang depending on the person's constitution. And finally, I will share the whole life diet, which is the balanced diet for someone who is healthy to maintain their health.

So who is the immune diet for? Everyone! Well, 60–70 percent of the population will need this diet. The food we eat lowers our immune system, breathing poor quality air or through a mask lowers our immune system, and even our attitudes, emotions, and the "stress of life" lowers our immune system.

Sadly, they did not teach us proper nutrition in medical school. One thing I learned is this: The ones entrusted with healing people are not taught proper nutrition. Rather, they learn only to recognize the disease and prescribe a pill to hopefully remedy it, without even considering a change to the lifestyle.

The immune system is a cooperating life force that enables you to integrate the outside with the inside. This is based on the ability to maintain good bacteria; it provides you with the ability to adapt to your environment.

This adaptive ecosystem within you helps you to develop immunity to what you come in contact with. Microbes are important life forms, which are harmonious with you. It is important to understand that every external membrane of your body has microbes. When I say external, I mean every surface (skin, lungs, intestinal tract, and urinary tract) that can be touched without piercing the body. The microbes are like a force field that protects you. These microbes will perform digestive functions and produce preventative by-products to help you. In performing their duties, they get to live if you have good parameters for them to thrive. It is called the terrain, which is the food you eat. There are other factors such as emotions and activities that affect the body's pH and the motility of the digestive system. Chemicals are the most detrimental and injurious to this terrain. This terrain or another way to put it is liquid nutrient solution "chime" changes the ability of the microbes, or "the good bacteria," to grow. When you have the correct factors, you will grow only the good bacteria. When you have the incorrect factors, the bad bacteria, mold, yeasts, and fungus will grow.

The ability to have the proper nutrients, which enables you to grow good bacteria, will keep you healthy. The immune diet is all based on that.

If you recall, I mentioned earlier that the nutrient chi sponsors the immune chi. The better you can digest food and have it mix well with the good bacteria, the better the intestines will grow good bacteria. Eighty-five percent of your immune system is a result of the beneficial bacteria that is in your gut, or better said, your intestinal tract.

As a repeat from previously in the book, I want to emphasize the importance of having a beneficial bacterial condition on all the external membranes of the body; this is the critical factor in one's health. Like in compost, the bacteria break the food down into recyclable nutrients. Your intestine does this function for you so that the chime is in a state that will enable the body's enzymes to change the nutrients into absorbable nutrients that are able to enter your blood. You have your own personal yogurt factory in your intestinal tract! One of the main by-products of the bacteria growing is a waste called *hydrogen peroxide*. When hydrogen peroxide comes in contact with anaerobic bacteria, it will kill the bad bacteria as well as molds, yeasts, and fungus. Processed foods and chemicals, especially Roundup, will kill the good bacteria. All around the world, humans have always had some form of bacteria in their diet in the form of fermented foods that they have eaten regularly to maintain better health. There are 100 trillion good bacteria in the healthy gut, which is more than cells in your body. Be nice to them as they are your best friends! Now you know what I mean by the saying, "Every culture has its culture!"

Now that you have the concept of how the immune system is maintained, it is up to you to know where you are daily and what you need to do to maintain your healthy gut—how you eat, rest, exercise, and think, as well as environmental factors. The daily routines are called a **lifestyle**! Your lifestyle will determine what bacteria will grow: good versus bad. Your gut-brain connection is critical to the state of your health and your moods and attitudes. If it is damaged at a young age, it will have an impact on your mental development. Chemicals are the primary cause of childhood mental disorders, especially glyphosate, antibiotics, and vaccines. They kill your good bacteria and put chemicals into the body. These chemicals include concentrated "vitamins." Do realize vitamin tablets are man-made chemicals and are too concentrated for good bacteria to grow on.

The most important food to have when you are critically sick is chicken broth-base soups with stalk and root vegetables along with sea salts and fifteen drops of ConcenTrace mineral drops added to the soup bowl. This will provide the nutrient chi to restart your parameters or the good stuff to set your body right, so only the good bacteria will grow. Chicken will raise your body temperature, vegetables will give you bulk and energy to allow the good bacteria to grow, and sea salts and ConcenTrace provide the alkalinity from the minerals such as zinc. Krill oil will give you the vitamin D3. Oregano oil is the hottest herb and has antimicrobial properties.

Probiotics give you a restart to the good gut bacteria. Soup and teas will hydrate you and provide the yang to remedy the extreme yin. The important thing is to establish a more alkaline state, as only good bacteria can live in this condition. Sunlight and fresh air are important when you are out of the crisis.

THE FIVE AREAS WHERE YOU SPEND YOUR ENERGY OR "CHI"

1. Digesting food
2. Physical activity
3. Mental activity
4. Reproducing yourself
5. Healing yourself

When you are healthy, the body can juggle all five of these functions, but when you are sick, you need to stop doing the extra things that drain your energy or chi. You need to have foods that are easy to digest along with rest. When you are sick, you do not have the energy to digest food. The most extreme case of this is when you go into a coma; you shut down everything except the healing of the body. This is a weakened state (too yin), and you will need to have cooked light warming and alkalizing foods that hydrate you along with not spending any of your energy on physical activities. In the case of most flus and colds, your acute immune problems will respond quickly in days. Let your energy levels be your guide to expanding more food choices and activities. As you improve, add organic brown rice to the soup for more glucose that aids in the ability to grow more good bacteria; also add chicken meat for protein to give you the yangizing "strengthening" effect.

To understand your immune system, you should observe your feces—no other way to put it. Notice the nature of the feces as to its regularity, amount, shape, smell, buoyancy, and form. This will tell you how your bacteria in your intestinal lining were doing earlier in the day or the previous day.

The following description will require you to look in the toilet once your job is done, so please try not to be grossed out!

The feces should be firm-looking and shaped like a banana. There should be no bad odor. Bad odor is a sign that you may be having trouble in either the stomach or the intestines.

If your feces are light in color, then you are more yin. If your feces are darker, you are yang and eating heavy foods such as animal products or processed foods. Normal feces should be brown. If the feces sink to the bottom of the toilet, you have been eating the wrong type of foods or you are not taking the time to eat properly (you are eating on the run and not chewing your foods). When you eat good quality foods and you properly chew your foods, the feces should remain on the surface.

In the case of an infant, the baby feces should be yellow and somewhat soft. If the feces are brown, the baby is getting too yang quality of foods. When a newborn baby feces is green, the infant is not being given the proper foods, or the mother's milk is of poor quality (then the mother is too yin).

Other things we can learn from the feces: If you consume too much salt, the feces will be dryer; on the other hand, if you are eating mostly milk, fruits, and sugar and have an insufficient amount of salt in the foods, the feces will have no shape. Constipation is a yang presentation, and is brought on by things such as refined foods. The feces will be darker, rounder, and shinier in appearance. In some cases, there is a yin constipation—the stools are small and ball like, kind of like a rabbit turd but not shiny. It should be noted that the yin person should not take a laxative.

While your urine will tell you of more recent conditions, your stools will tell you more of the past few days.

ADVICE FROM MY HEALTHY DAD

I have used this principle for almost fifty years with thousands of excellent results. Trust nature and common sense. The old adage, "Starve a cold and drown a fever" is a truism! The pandemic is not as serious as it is made up to be once you understand these principles. Oxygen and alkalinity are the most important factors to health. Alkalinity maintains the red blood cells' ability to bind and carry oxygen by the red blood cells. There is no need for ventilators, which injure the lung's ability to get oxygen into the blood. The ventilators stress the lung by putting so much pressure on the tissue that it reduces the ability to transfer oxygen into the blood. It also dries out the lungs, thus reducing the moist environment, which is also a key element in transferring oxygen into the blood stream.

The goal is to have a long and healthy life, and if you maintain a quality lifestyle, you will have one. Disease is an imbalance of nature, so to understand nature, you will need to observe a continuum of a thousand years to see the cause and effect. Ageless wisdom will provide you with this. Knowing these principles will guide you through your life. Take the time to invest in your life, take the time to read the material that has worked and been around for over 4,000 years. The simplest one is yin and yang. Refer to Chapter 3 and the chart in the following section.

WHAT ARE THE SIGNS OF YIN AND YANG PATTERNS?

Here are some descriptions on signs of yin and yang patterns to look for when observing another individual.

DESCRIPTION	YIN	YANG
Looking	Quiet, withdrawn, guilty, frail, slow mannered, likes to lie down and curl up. No spirit, secretions are watery and thin. Tongue presentation is puffy, pale, and moist with white moss-like texture.	Loud, agitated, restless, active, rapid, forceful movements, reddish complexion, person would like to stretch when lying down. Tongue material is reddish and dry with yellowing thick moss-like nature.
Listening/Sound	Voice is low and without strength, few words, weak shallow respiration, and shortness of breath.	Loud voice is coarse, rough, and strong. Patient is talkative, respiration is full, strong, and deep.
Smell/Odor	Acrid odor, vegetable adrenal.	Putrid odor, sweaty smell.
Asking/Comments	Feels cool to cold, reduced appetite, no taste, warmth and touch, copious and clear urine.	Feels warm to hot, dislikes heat or touch, desires, constipation, dark scanty urine, dry mouth and thirst.
Touching/Feel	Frail, thin, empty, or weak.	Full, big rapid, slippery, wirier, floating, and strong.

INTRODUCTION TO THE IMMUNE DIET

In nature when things are balanced, there is no disease. The remaining portion of this chapter is the actual immune diet. It will be a guide to you to help you understand what foods are important and good, and what foods are poor and what you should avoid. When I give this to my patients who want to build their immune system, I tell them to keep it simple, pick and choose something in each category to either add or subtract from their current ways of eating. Over time, you will notice your body responding, and before you know it, you will be ready to jump into the whole life diet as explained in Chapter 11. You will still continue to apply the principles you learned in the immune diet, but it will now be a way of life for the rest of your life. You will "live it" through a lifestyle and you won't need to keep jumping on the fad diets.

IMMUNE DIET

The main goal of the immune diet is to reestablish the good digestive bacteria and provide help to your immune system. This diet will be based on individual needs, so it is important to know where your health resides at the present time.

The immune diet is designed for the short-term fix. This immune diet is recommended for people who currently fall in the category of –3 to –6 on the yin-yang scale. The goal is to get you between a –3 and a +3 on the yin-yang scale. Once you get between –3 and 3, you would switch to the whole life diet. The whole life diet, or what I would call the live-it lifestyle diet, is a way-of-life diet to help you on the course to a healthy retirement planning.

When you approach this diet, in each category you will see multiple items to choose from. It is my recommendation to choose one thing that you want from each area on the list and do the daily recommended serving.

Here are the subheadings for each category. It is important to follow these as outlined. It is assumed when I mention anything in the important and good sections that these items are organic, and those items in the avoid section contain GMO and GMF items.

- **IMPORTANT:** It's just that! It is important you follow and start implementing these food items into your daily regimen.
- **GOOD:** Does not have the same quality as the important ones, but it does have good qualities you will want to also

incorporate into your diet. The items listed under "good" give you more latitude for what to eat and drink.

- **POOR:** Is better than the avoid but not as good as those items listed in the good sections.
- **AVOID:** It's just that! Avoid at all measures. Avoiding these foods will help you transition to the whole life diet as most of the avoids in the whole life diet are also the same with a few variants.
- **COMMENTS:** This section will be listed at the bottom of each category and will give you greater insights.

I have simplified this diet because everyone is on a different level. This is only a quick reference guide. You can go to www. liveitlifestyles.com and print out a copy for yourself.

FERMENTED FOODS AND PROBIOTICS
Important

- Probiotics: Acidophilus, 5 billion active CFU/g in the refrigerator section of the store. Take 2 capsules 2–4 times a day.
- Fermented Foods: Sauerkraut, kimchi, cabbage, turnips, onions, and cucumbers
- Seaweeds: Wakame, dulse, kelp, kombu, nori, hijiki, agar agar, arame, bladderwrack, Irish moss, ogonori, and mozuku

Good

- Fermented Foods: Organic carrots, miso, tamari, tempeh, natto

Avoid

- Soy Foods: Soy milk, soybean oil, soy flour soy breads, edamame (raw soybeans in the pod), and tofu

- Take 2 capsules of acidophilus (probiotics) 2–4 times a day. Reduce to 1 time a day as you are doing better.
- It is best to take the acidophilus/probiotics at least 30–45 minutes or more before meals.
- A good brand of probiotics will have 5 billion active CFU/g and be found in the refrigerator section of the store.
- Probiotics will give you the restart to the good gut bacteria.

OILS, REFINED OILS, AND FRIED FOODS
Important

- Oils: Krill oil
- Omega-3 Oils: Skate oil, salmon oil, cod liver oils, Organic Valley and Kerrygold butters
- Essential Oils: Oregano oil

Poor

- Olive oil, coconut oil

Avoid

- Canola oil, soybean oil, hydrogenated oils, shortening, lard, oleo, margarine, bacon grease
- Deep-fried foods such as french fries, onion rings, nuts, corn chips, potato chips, tempura, chicken, fish
- Fatty food such as hamburgers, hot dogs, luncheon meats, sausage, and bacon

Comments

- Take 1–2 of the 350 mg krill oil capsules 2 times a day. Costco has the best quality and least expensive option, called Kirkland krill oil.

- Omega-3 oils: use at least 1–2 tablespoons each day using 100% grass-fed butter or fish liver oil.
- Essential oregano oil: Take 2–5 drops 2–4 times a day after meals when you have congestion or bloating, then reduce to 1–2 times a day as you are doing better.
- Do not take oregano oil straight but dilute it with four parts of olive oil to one part oregano oil.
- If you have congestion, use an atomizer at night in the bedroom with 10 drops of 100% oregano oil.
- Krill oil will give you vitamin D3 and oregano oil is the hottest herb and has antimicrobial properties.

BEVERAGES, MINERALS, STIMULANTS, ALCOHOL, AND TEAS

Important

- Beverage: Reverse osmosis (RO) water is best
- Minerals: ConcenTrace minerals

Good

- Herb teas: Rooibos, raspberry, cleavers, chamomile, cherry bark, ginger, dandelion, ginseng
- Juices: Unsweetened cranberry, pomegranate, blueberry, and cherry
- Herb Root Teas: Echinacea, licorice, astragalus, dandelion, and burdock root

Avoid

- Stimulants: Caffeine, coffee, black and green teas, chocolate,

cocoa, cola drinks, energy drinks, NoDoz, Excedrin, cocaine, amphetamines
- Alcohol: Beer, wine, liquor
- Teas: Black teas, including morning thunder, guarana mate, black mountain, earl grey, and kali tea

Comments

- ConcenTrace minerals: Take 10–15 drops 2–4 times a day in at least 4 ounces of liquid or soup.
- Watch your urine. If it has too much color all day, you will need to drink more, but if you are clear, drink less.
- Herb Teas: Drink 2–4 cups a day. Directions: Use ¼ teaspoon of each herb for 1–2 of the teas to be made. Bring the water to a boil, then put the herbs into the hot water. Simmer roots with lid on for 15 minutes or steep leaves for 3 minutes.
- Most noncaffeine herbs are good.

FRUITS, VEGETABLES, SWEETS, AND SUGARS

Important

- Dark Greens: Bok choy, dandelion, kale, collard, seaweed
- Stalk Vegetables: Asparagus, broccoli, celery, leeks, green beans
- Root Vegetables: Dandelion, burdock, onions, rutabagas, turnips, radishes
- Salt: Very good quality of sea salt is important
- Spices: Cinnamon, cilantro, chives, ginger, garlic, oregano, thyme, basil, seaweeds
- Fermented Vegetables: Sauerkraut, kimchi, cabbage, turnips, onions, cucumbers
- Seaweeds: Wakame, dulse, kelp, kombu nori, hijiki, agar, arame, bladderwrack, Irish moss

- Fruits: Grapefruit, the juice and the pulp
- Berries: Blueberries

Good

- Dark Greens: Beets, mustard greens, chard, spinach
- Stalk Vegetables: Brussels sprouts, cauliflower, cabbage
- Root Vegetables: Carrots, parsnips, beets
- Fruits: Lemons, limes
- Berries: Most berries

Poor

- Vegetables: Sweet corn
- Sugar: Stevia

Avoid

- Nightshade Vegetables: Tomatoes, potatoes, eggplant, chilis, peppers
- Fruits and Fruit Juices: Orange, tangerine, pineapple, grape, apple, pear, mango, dried fruits
- Natural Sweeteners: Raw cane sugar, dates, honey, molasses, agave and maple syrups
- Beverages: Soda pop (both diet and regular), natural or regular fruit juice, Gatorade, sports drinks, energy drinks, all alcohol
- Sugars: White sugar, sucrose, high-fructose corn syrup, sweeteners
- Artificial Sugars: Saccharin, NutraSweet, aspartame, Splenda, sucralose
- Sweets: Candies, cookies, cakes, ice cream, fruit yogurts, fruit rollups, jams, jelly, Jell-O puddings

Comments

- Have ¼ to ½ cup of blueberries a day especially cooked in oatmeal. Oatmeal with blueberries is best in the morning and can even be used as an evening treat.
- It is important that you have 2–4 servings a day of vegetables whether in fermented form, soup, stew, stir-fry, casserole, or baked. Steamed vegetables are good. Use organic beef or chicken stock to make the soup or stew and eat at least a cup with each meal.
- Barley and malt syrups are okay but of poor quality, as they are in the glucose category.
- Don't have foods if they are raw or cold, and best not to have leftovers that are over 2 days old.
- **COOK ALL YOUR FOODS AND CHEW VERY WELL FOR BEST DIGESTION!**
- Look in sauces and drinks for anything that has high-fructose corn syrup and sweeteners and avoid them.

PROTEINS: VEGETABLES AND ANIMALS, BEANS AND LEGUMES

- Have 1–2 servings a day of vegetable proteins.
- Have 1–3 servings of 4–8 ounces of animal proteins a day.

Important

- Vegetable Protein: Spirulina
- Fowl: Cage-free chicken, turkey, eggs
- Fish: Wild-caught salmon, halibut, sea bass
- Beef: 100% grass-fed beef

Good

- Vegetable Proteins: Nuts and seeds, mung beans, brown rice, snow peas
- Dairy: Butter
- Animal Proteins: Lamb, pork, wild game
- Fish: Tuna, shark marlin, swordfish, pike, walleye, shrimp (see comments)

Avoid

- Animal Proteins: Farm-raised fish, grain-fed beef, caged chicken
- GMO Dairy Products: Milk, cheeses, cream, sour cream, ice cream, kefir, yogurt
- Vegetable Proteins: Soybeans, lentils, peas, lima beans

Comments

- Beans and legumes are hard to digest.
- Eat only 100% grass-fed beef!
- Have cilantro and fermented vegetables to detoxify the mercury that is found in fish.

100% WHOLE GRAIN, REFINED GRAINS, SNACK FOODS, AND YEAST-CONTAINING FOODS

- Have 1–2 serving a day of 100% whole grains in cooked cereals or casseroles.

Important

- Grains: Organic brown rice, oatmeal, quinoa, spelt

Good

- Grains: Organic millet, barley, buckwheat, rye, triticale

Poor

- Grains: 100% whole wheat pasta and toasted sprouted bread, corn

Avoid

- GMO soy and corn
- Refined Grains: White flour, unbleached flour, cracked wheat, most bread, pasta, pizza crust, pretzels, cereals, crackers
- 100% Whole Grain: All wheat flour products unless labeled whole wheat
- Snack Foods: Cakes doughnuts, cookies
- Yeast-Containing Foods: Baking and nutritional brewer's yeasts and autolyzed yeast

Comments

- When making casseroles, cooked grains, or cereals, make sure to use organic ingredients.
- Eat only organic corn products; soy and corn are always GMO.
- If you have congestion, do not eat flour products such as wheat, buckwheat, rye, corn, and triticale.

SAUCES, SOY FOODS, CHEMICALS, AND DRUGS
Good

- Soy Foods: Fermented organic soy such as miso and tamari

Avoid

- Soy Foods: Soymilk, soybean oil, soy flour and breads, edamame (raw soybeans in the pod)
- Sauces: Ketchup, most dressings and sauces like Worcestershire, Chinese plum, teriyaki, and sweet and sour
- Drugs: NSAIDS (Ibuprofen, Motrin, Aleve, Advil, Tylenol, aspirin)
- Chemicals: Endocrine disrupters, steroids, antibiotics, HRT, HGH growth hormones, preservatives, flavor agents, MSG, glutamate, autolyzed yeast, casein, caseinate commercial soup, broth, and sauces
- GMO and GMF genetically modified organism or foods: Soy, corn, sugar beets, canola oil, cotton seed oil
- Sauces: Hot sauces, salsas, red curry, spaghetti sauce

Comments

- Most sauces have MSG in them if they say hydrolyzed vegetable proteins (HVP) or texturized vegetable proteins (TVP).
- HRT, HGH growth hormones, steroids, and antibiotics are given to the animals or put in milk; these are also known as endocrine disrupters and will have a very bad effect on the immune system and promote excessive cell growth.
- Avoid most vitamins and pills if called health products, as they are just chemicals and you do not need them.
- Generally, steamed foods are poor if you have a lot of phlegm.

GENERAL INFORMATION

- The most important food to have when you are critically sick is chicken broth-base soups with stalk and root vegetables along with sea salt. Add 15 drops of ConcenTrace mineral drops to a bowl. This will provide the nutrient chi to restart your parameters, the good stuff to set your body right so only the good bacteria will grow. Chicken will raise your body temperature, vegetables will give you bulk and energy for the bacteria to grow, and sea salt along with ConcenTrace provide the alkalinity from the minerals like zinc.

- Don't eat raw or cold foods. Do not have leftover foods of more than a day old as they may develop mold or bacteria in them.
- Avoid microwave devices especially at night, cell phones and remote phones, Wi-Fi, 5G, smart meters, and blue lights.
- Avoid overdoing things like exercising, working, eating, worrying, thinking, and staying up too late at night.
- Avoid drafty rooms and getting chilled and cold feet. It is good to wear shoes and socks.
- To prevent getting chilled, dry your hair before going to bed so there is no wet hair on the neck or ears.
- Stay warm and dry. Get sunlight and movement.
- Read the labels of the things you buy. If you see words or names that you cannot pronounce or recognize, you know it is not good for you.

HOW HAVE I APPLIED THE IMMUNE DIET IN MY CLINICAL PRACTICE?

One of the most important diets is the immune diet. In my practice, when I see fungal toenails, the first thing that comes to mind is, this person's immune system is off. I first ask when they injured the nail. Then they respond that they either dropped something on their toe or were wearing a tight pair of shoes. Then I pose a different question to them: How is it that you can injure one toe, and then months or years later you see the fungus appear on the toes of the opposite foot? It is because the fungus is in our bloodstream. It is an internal factor. We all have fungus in our system, but when our body cannot fight off the excessive fungus, we start to develop more fungus, which is commonly expressed in the toenails. In order to really get rid of the fungus, we have to jump-start the immune system. We must establish good bacteria through the nutrition mix, lay off the sugars, eat real foods, and be aware of junk oils, along with proper rest and diet.

One thing I will add to this discussion is if you have a fungal infection in your toes, start soaking your toes in a gallon of warm water with 2 tablespoons of baking soda for ten minutes at least three times a week. Along with this diet, I have seen some amazing changes.

CONCLUSION

If 60–70 percent of the people today are in need of an immune boost, I cannot think of a better way than this simple immune diet to start. In today's world, everything has been chemicalized from foods to the water we drink and even the air we breathe. We all need a daily boost to our immune system. Once your immune system is compromised, this is when you see your wealth go to your health. If we can slow that down or by having a strong immune system, you will be able to enjoy your retirement years. Coming from a doctor who treats patients, I can tell you that your immune system is so precious. Guard it with your life and you will be making fewer trips to the doctor's office. You cannot put a price on your health!

There are many ways the body will tell you if your immune system is off. The main one I will point out aside from fungal toenails is the common cold with flu-like symptoms. How often do you run to the urgent care or doctor's office to get an antibiotic?

In Chapter 10, you will be introduced to the diabetic diet. If you don't have diabetes, you may want to skip to Chapter 11 where I introduce the whole life diet or, as I call it, the "live-it lifestyle." When someone has seen the benefits of the immune diet, this is the diet I will gravitate them toward unless there is something else that may need to be addressed.

The immune diet is the yin diet. The diabetic diet is more of the yang diet. The whole life diet is the balancer; it is what I do on a daily basis along with the nutrient mix detox.

CHAPTER 10

Don't Let a Crisis Go to Your Waist

The Live-It Lifestyle for the Diabetic Diet

———

If you are one of the 34.2 million people who are suffering from diabetes in the United States or the 425 million diabetics in the world, this chapter is for you. If you have a relative or friend who has diabetes, this chapter is for you. If you have been told you are pre-diabetic, this chapter is for you. From what we learned in Chapter 3, you will see there is actually a yin diabetic and a yang diabetic and they are treated differently. This chapter will also explore other means to reducing your blood sugars other than foods.

Diabetes is hereditary only because you ate the way your parents did. Because you eat the way your society (family, friends, and environment) trained you, you did not know the difference. Your pancreas, this special organ, gets tired from having only sugar or too much sugar. It's like if you ran a marathon and never took the time to sleep. You would have to stop running the marathons because your body would break down. Diabetes is no different from getting the common cold. Your body is run down, you're exhausted, and your immune system is now not working to its full potential.

How do diabetes and your immune system work together? Your immune system is based on self-esteem (emotions) and poor food choices (biology). Your self-esteem is vital when you don't feel loved or wanted. I will even take it a step further. If you don't follow the third great commandment, "The Ability to Love Yourself," this will greatly affect your diabetes. Low self-esteem, or an inability to love yourself, is a factor for diabetes. If you have too much worry, you're going to eat too much sugar. That is why it is called comfort food. It's a temporary fix for the present situation.

WHAT DO YOU MEAN BY PLACATE?

When you are conscious or present, you will be healthier. You will start to say I'm going to get some rest. I'm not going to have those foods with bad chemicals. Diabetes is nothing more than a chemical imbalance that is demanding the blood sugar so high that your insulin can't produce enough to keep up with your present eating habits or emotional situations. The proof is being expressed physically now. If you don't change the diet and don't lower the sugars by eating long-term fuel instead of short-term fuel, the pancreas cannot catch up. You won't have to have insulin.

WHAT IS THE DIFFERENCE BETWEEN TYPE 1 AND TYPE 2 DIABETES?

Type 2 diabetes is directly a result from your lifestyle (foods and emotions). Type 2 diabetes sees the pancreas as the source of help, The pancreas wants help to produce more insulin to help the high sugar levels in the body. Type 1 diabetes is an auto-immune disorder; it is where your pancreas is being attacked because the body recognizes the pancreas as the problem.

Responding to the current discussion, I related this experience to my Healthy Dad. Back in 2012, I met a lady who was a salesperson for a company that designed a gadget that could be placed on the abdomen of a person, and with a small needle, the device would connect to the inner area of the stomach region with no pain. The device would then register with a handheld device that would show you your active sugar levels. I asked to volunteer for a two-week experimental experience for myself. These devices are readily available now, but back then they were only reserved for the Type 1 diabetic. The device was attached to my lower abdominal area; a protective film was used to cover the device so I could still take showers and work out.

Once I got the device, I experimented with it. I ate pizza and noticed my sugar level rise. The more slices of pizza, the more it climbed, and it remained high for several hours. I also ate things that I have been telling my patients to eat for years to help lower their blood sugar; the big three were blueberries, green beans, and ginger root.

The blueberries slowly lowered my blood sugar. The green beans also lowered my blood sugars. Then it came down with the ginger root. Since I was not advanced in preparing my meals with ginger, I decided to just take a bite of ginger. *I don't recommend this!* What I noted with the straight ginger aside from my tongue being on fire was something amazing. It lowered my blood sugar very fast just like insulin would do to a diabetic. It went so fast that it was a bit scary.

I even took this test a step further. I lay down in a quiet place, took a reading of my sugars, and recorded it. I then used my mind to create a sad story in my head. I thought about how I missed my children and how I felt that nobody really loved or appreciated me. As I played out these stories, I was amazed that my blood sugar level was rising just like when I ate the pizza. To protect myself, I did everything to change that story in my head and started to create a story of feeling loved, appreciated, and a feeling of high self-worth. To my surprise, my blood sugar numbers started to fall.

YIN DIABETIC AND YANG DIABETIC

Here are some simple guidelines with diabetes. Most diabetics are yin (weak, tired, stressed), so cooking your food is the best way to eat prepared meals. There are those who are yang (strong, hot, energized). They will do best with more raw foods. The key factor in understanding if you are yin or yang is to ask yourself this question: Am I cold or hot? Am I always pulling the covers over me, or am I kicking the covers off? This is very important because if you are weak, tired, and have no strength and if you are eating raw, you are only going to make yourself weaker and more tired. On the other hand, if you are strong, hot, and energized, that grass-fed beef steak may not be the right choice. You will do better with the rawer foods. So whether you are yin or yang, start with eating unprocessed foods: fresh vegetables, whole grains, and quality animal foods as mentioned above. Eat veggies prepared this way. The more yang you are, eat rawer; the more yin you are, then slightly cook your food. The concept is to cook the food so that there is still a great deal of texture in the foods.

WHY IS THE YANG DIABETIC MORE ASSOCIATED WITH THE HEART WHEREAS THE YIN DIABETIC IS ASSOCIATED WITH ILLNESSES AND INFECTIONS?

Sugars in all forms will be converted into fat if not metabolized quickly, as the blood cannot have sugar stay in the blood. This fat builds up interstitially in tissues and arteries of the body. This will cause a heart circulation problem resulting in blocked vessels. When I say sugars, I mean all sugars: syrups, sweets, candies, soda pop, sports drinks, most fruits, and white flour.

Another reason the heart gets a buildup of plaque in the arteries is that the acids inflame the interior blood vessel wall. The body will use cholesterol as a healing solvent to cover the inflammation. The interior blood vessel wall gets a stretch mark that makes a rough surface or gets inflamed and that causes turbulence in the blood flow. This is of major consequence as you cannot have a whirlpool effect in the blood because it will cause the red blood cells to stick together and form a clot. The body's natural ability to survive this is to put cholesterol over the rough surface to decrease the turbulence and lower the clotting propensity. Clots are the cause of strokes and blood circulation in the legs or in more severe cases into the lungs. When one is not treated soon, it will cause death by a pulmonary embolism.

It is important to reduce the acids in the blood to prevent heart disease caused by arterial plaque buildup. These acid substances in your blood are insulin, sugar, homocysteine, lactic acid, uric acid, purines, bilirubin, and cortisol, which is also known as stress hormone or adrenaline.

Diabetes usually goes with or comes before heart disease, so watch the alcohol, sugars, and high-fructose corn syrup.

DIABETIC DIET

The diabetic diet is designed to help the yin presentations (feeling weak, tired, and cold) and for the yang presentations (strong, hot) in balancing your blood sugars. Your constitution and how you apply this diet will determine how long you stay on this diet. Once your blood sugars are in the normal range, then you may switch over to the whole life diet. It is my recommendation to work closely with your primary care doctor as the things I suggest here will lower your blood sugars. If you are on insulin, it is vital you watch your blood sugars and adjust your insulin accordingly with the guidance of your physician.

When you approach this diet, in each category you will see multiple items to choose from. It is my recommendation to choose one thing that you want from each area on the list and do the daily recommended serving.

Here are the subheading for each category, and it is important to follow these as outlined. It is assumed when I mention anything in the important and good sections, these items are organic, and those items in the avoid section contain GMO and GMF items.

- **IMPORTANT:** Is just that! It is important you follow and start implementing these food items into your daily regimen.
- **GOOD:** Does not have the quality as the important ones, but it does have the good qualities you will want to also incorporate; it gives you more latitude for what to eat and drink.
- **POOR:** Is better than the avoid but not as good as those items listed in the good section.
- **AVOID:** It's just that! Avoid at all measures. Avoiding these foods will help you transition to the whole life diet as most of the avoids in the whole life diet are also the same with a few variants.

- **COMMENTS:** This section will be listed at the bottom of each category and will give you greater insights.

I have simplified this diet because everyone is on a different level. This is only a quick reference guide. You can go to www.liveitlifestyles.com and print out a copy for yourself.

INSULIN-LOWERING FOODS

- Ginger, cinnamon, cloves, green beans, blueberries, Jerusalem artichokes, or sun chokes
- Coconut oil and Kerrygold butter, also pure cod liver oil; use 1–2 tablespoons of each every day.
- Fresh ginger juice: Take 1 teaspoon in a ½ cup of warm water 2–4 times a day; it is best to take before each meal.
- The best way to make the juice is to finely grate about 1 tablespoon of the raw fresh ginger, then put in a garlic press and squeeze out a teaspoon of fresh juice. Cheese cloth also works.
- This will lower the need for insulin, so test yourself regularly to be sure you do not take too much insulin.

FERMENTED FOODS AND PROBIOTICS
Comments

- Take 2 capsules of acidophilus (probiotics) 1–2 times a day, then reduce to 1 time a day as you are doing better. It is best to take at least 30–45 minutes or more before meals.
- A good brand of probiotics will have 5 billion active CFU/g that is found in the refrigerator section of the store.

OILS, REFINED OILS, AND FRIED FOODS

Important

- Krill oil, skate oil, salmon oil, cod liver oil, Organic Valley and Kerrygold butter, and 100% grass-fed animal fats.

Good

- Coconut and olive oil are good.

Avoid

- Grain-fed animal fats, hydrogenated oils, shortening, lard, margarine, bacon grease, and refined oils especially canola oil and soybean oil.
- Deep-fried foods such as french fries, onion rings, nuts, corn chips, potato chips, tempura, chicken, fish. Fatty foods such as hamburgers, hot dogs, luncheon meats, sausage, and bacon.

Comments

- Take krill oil, 2 of the 350-mg capsules 2–4 times a day. Costco has the best quality and least expensive called Kirkland krill oil.
- Omega-3 oils: Use at least 2–6 tablespoons each day using 100% grass-fed butter or fish liver oil.

BEVERAGES, MINERALS, STIMULANTS, ALCOHOL, AND TEAS

- Drink 2–4 cups a day of herb teas such as ginger, cinnamon, and blueberry.

Important

- Reverse osmosis water with ConcenTrace minerals is best

Good

- Water, vegetable juice, and herb teas. Most noncaffeine herbs are good.
- Herb Teas: Rooibos, cleavers ginger root, dandelion root, burdock root, yellow dock root, echinacea, ginger burdock, and sarsaparilla
- Juices: Unsweetened cranberry, blueberry, and cherry

Avoid

- Caffeine, coffee, green teas, beer, wine, liquor
- Teas: Black tea, morning thunder, guarana mate, black mountain, earl grey, kali tea, green tea
- Stimulants: Chocolate, cocoa, cola drinks, energy drinks, NoDoz, Excedrin, cocaine, amphetamines

Comments

- Watch your urine; if it has too much color all day, you will need to drink more, but if your urine is clear, drink less.
- Herb Tea: Directions: Use ½ teaspoon of each herb for 1–3 cups of tea to be made. Bring the water to a boil, then put the herbs into the water and simmer roots for 15 minutes or steep leaves for 3–5 minutes.
- The best root teas are echinacea, licorice, astragalus, dandelion, and burdock root. Most noncaffeine herbs are good.
- It is important to chew all your food very well for best digestion.
- ConcenTrace Minerals: Take 10–15 drops 2–4 times a day in at least 4 ounces of liquid or soup.

FRUITS, VEGETABLES, SWEETS, AND SUGARS

- Vegetables: 2–4 servings a day either fermented, salad, juice, soup, stew, stir-fry, steamed, casserole, or baked
- Fruits: ¼–½ cup a day. All berries, especially blueberries

Important

- Salad Greens: Romaine, red left, bib, arugula, spring mix, to name a few
- Dark Greens: bok choy, dandelion, kale, collard, romaine and lettuces, beet, mustard, chard greens, and spinach
- Stalk: Asparagus, broccoli, celery, leeks, green beans
- Root: Carrots, dandelion, burdock, onions, parsnips, rutabagas, turnips, radishes
- Spices: Cinnamon, cilantro, chives, ginger, garlic, oregano, thyme, basil
- Salad Dressing: Olive oil, mustard, lemon and lime juices, balsamic and apple cider, and vinegar and blend with any herbs
- Salts: Very good quality sea salt is important
- Fermented: Sauerkraut and kimchi, cabbage, turnips, carrots, onions, cucumbers

Good

- Dark Greens: Beets, mustard, chard, spinach
- Stalk: Brussels sprouts, cauliflower, cabbage
- Root: Beets
- Salts: Tamari, miso; use in small amounts and is best to cook into the food
- Fermented: Miso, tamari, tempeh, natto
- Fruits: Grapefruit, lemon, lime, all berries, cherries

Poor

- Sweet corn
- Stevia
- Natural Sweeteners: Barley and malt are okay syrups

Avoid

- Nightshade vegetables such as tomatoes, potatoes, eggplant, chilis, peppers
- All Fruits and Juices: Orange, tangerine, pineapple, grape, apple, mango, pear, peach, apricot, plum, and dried fruit
- Natural Sweeteners: Raw cane, date, honey, molasses, agave, maple
- Beverages: Soda pop (diet or regular), natural or regular fruit juice, Gatorade, sports drinks, energy drinks, all alcohol
- Sugars: White, sucrose, high-fructose corn syrup, sweeteners
- Artificial Sugars: NutraSweet, aspartame, amino sweet, Neotame and Splenda, sucralose, and saccharin
- Sweets: Candies, cookies, cakes, ice cream, fruit yogurts, fruit rollups, jams, jelly, Jell-O puddings

Comments

- It is good to eat raw foods and vegetable juices if you do not have sinus or lung congestion or phlegm.
- Have ¼–½ cup of blueberries a day especially if cooked in oatmeal. Oatmeal with blueberries is best in the morning and can even be used as an evening treat.
- Look in sauces and drinks for anything that has high-fructose corn syrup and sweeteners and avoid them.

PROTEINS: VEGETABLES AND ANIMALS

- Vegetables: 1–2 serving a day
- Animal: Have a 4–8 ounce serving 4–6 times a week (soup or stew is best)

Important

- Mung beans and brown rice
- Spirulina, bee pollen, nuts and seeds
- Free-range chicken, turkey, lean beef, and eggs
- Wild game and eggs with soft yolks only
- Wild-caught salmon, halibut
- Grass-fed beef

Good

- Some goat or sheep yogurt and soft white cheese such as feta are okay, but only for flavor.
- Pork
- High-Mercury Fish: Tuna, shark, sea bass, marlin, swordfish, pike, walleye

Poor

- Mexican oysters

Avoid

- Unnaturally raised animals: Chicken, farm-raised fish, corn-fed animals, and generally animals that are not raised in a natural environment.
- All dairy products unless 100% grass-fed

Comments

- If you eat fish regularly, eat ½ bunch of cilantro with fish to detoxify the mercury.

100% WHOLE GRAIN, REFINED GRAINS, SNACK FOODS, AND YEAST-CONTAINING FOODS

- 1–3 servings a day. Cook grains, cereals, and casseroles.

Important

- Organic brown rice, oatmeal, quinoa, spelt, millet, barley, buckwheat

Good

- Wheat, rye, triticale

Poor

- Corn

Avoid

- GMO soy and corn
- All wheat flour products unless it says organic whole wheat, white flour, unbleached flour, cracked wheat, most bread, pasta, pizza crust, pretzels, cereals, crackers, cakes, doughnuts, cookies. Corn products unless organic.

Comments

- When making casseroles, cooked grains, or cereals, make sure to use organic ingredients.
- Eat only organic corn products; soy and corn are always GMO.
- Breads are good if you have no phlegm or congestion.
- If you have congestion, do not eat flour products such as wheat, buckwheat, rye, corn, and triticale.

SAUCES, SPICES, SALTS, AND CHEMICALS AND DRUGS
Important

- Cinnamon, cilantro, chives, ginger, garlic, oregano, thyme, basil, seaweeds
- Very good quality sea salt

Good

- Tamari, miso

Avoid

- Distilled vinegar, ketchup, most dressings and sauces such as Worcestershire, Chinese plum, teriyaki, and sweet and sour
- NSAIDS (Ibuprofen, Motrin, Aleve, Advil, Tylenol, aspirin)
- Endocrine disrupters, steroids, antibiotics, HRT, HGH growth hormones
- Preservatives, flavor agents, MSG, glutamate, autolyzed yeast, casein, caseinate, commercial soup, broth, and sauces
- GMO and GMF genetically modified organisms or foods such as soy, corn, sugar beets, canola oil, and cotton seed oils
- Hot sauces, salsas, red curry, spaghetti sauce
- No oil-soluble vitamins A and E, natural or synthetic

Comments

- Most sauces have MSG in them if they say hydrolyzed vegetable proteins (HVP) or texturized vegetable proteins (TVP).
- HRT, HGH growth hormones, steroids, and antibiotics are given to animals or put in milk. These are also known as endocrine disrupters and will have a very bad effect on the immune system and promote excessive cell growth.
- Avoid most vitamins and pills if called health products, as they are just chemicals and you do not need them.
- Generally, steamed foods are poor if you have a lot of phlegm.

COOLING AND SPICY FOODS
Avoid

- Nightshade vegetables such as tomatoes, potatoes, eggplant, peppers, chilis
- Hot sauces, red curry, peppermint, ketchup, spaghetti sauce

GENERAL INFORMATION

- Don't eat raw or cold foods. Do not have leftover foods of more than a day old, as they may develop mold or bacteria in them.
- Avoid microwave devices especially at night, cell phones and remote phones, Wi-Fi, 5G, smart meters, and blue lights.
- Avoid overdoing things such as exercising, working, eating, worrying, thinking, and staying up too late at night.
- Avoid drafty rooms and getting chilled and cold feet. It is good to wear shoes and socks.
- To prevent getting chilled, dry your hair before going to bed so there is no wet hair on the neck or ears.
- Stay warm and dry. Get sunlight and movement.
- Read the labels of the things you buy. If you see words or

names you cannot pronounce or recognize, you know it is not good for you.

IMPORTANT INFORMATION FOR BLOOD SUGAR AND DIABETIC PROBLEMS

Start with eating unprocessed food, fresh vegetables, whole grains, and quality animal foods as mentioned above.

Eat vegetables prepared this way: if you are more yang, have them raw; if you aremore yin , you will want to slightly cook them.

The concept is to cook the food so that there is still a great deal of texture still in the foods.

It is best to have food in this general proportion each day. Be sure to have them organic and GMO-free.

- 25%–30% whole grains and cereals cooked well; pressure cooking is best
- 35%–40% vegetables = 15% root, 20% stalk, and 5% leaf
- 20%–25% organic 100% grass-fed meats and dairy and non-GMO-fed animals: chicken, fish, and eggs
- 5%–8% beans and lentils
- 5%–8% nuts and seeds
- 3%–5% fermented foods, condiments, and spices

Eat these foods regularly, as they will help you best lower your blood sugars. Remember: It is important to watch your blood sugar regularly to be sure you don't take too much insulin.

- Cinnamon

- Ginger (fastest blood sugar reducer when it is taken fresh and raw in juice)
- Cloves
- Jerusalem artichokes or sun chokes
- Coconut
- Blueberries
- Green beans
- Buckwheat
- Short-grain organic Lundberg brown rice and all whole grains only
- Red lentils and adzuki beans
- Kudzu (thickening agent for sauces)
- Gomashio (80% ground and roasted seeds with some very high-quality sea salt)

Eat these foods regularly, as they will help you increase magnesium in your blood.

- Best ones: Kelp, dulse, and all seaweed
- Great ones: Almonds, cashews, brazil nuts, filberts, sesame seeds, peanuts, coconut, walnuts, avocados
- Very good ones: Greens, collards, kale, beets, spinach, turnips, cilantro, parsley
- Good ones: Whole wheat, millet, brown rice, rye lentils

Key lifestyle things to improve on:

- Drink only enough to have a color of real light yellowish to the urine.
- Chew your food exceptionally well so you drink your food.
- Eat roughage or bulk to slow down the absorption of carbohydrates and sugars.

- Include good bacteria daily from fermented foods and probiotics.
- Avoid soybeans, even organic, except organic non-GMO fermented miso and tamari or tempeh and natto.

WHAT HAVE I OBSERVED FROM THIS CHAPTER ON DIABETES?

Having been in practice for over twenty years, diabetes is one of those diseases that can be easily corrected through diet and loving yourself. When I work with a patient, I will work with them on what foods to avoid and help them understand there is nobody else like them in the world and that they are a very important piece to the puzzle in the human race. If they truly want to participate in the process, amazing things happen.

You literally are what you eat. I have seen patients who are pre-diabetic, meaning they are not yet put on medication to control their blood sugars. Once they change their eating habits, they see their blood sugars come down. I have seen patients with levels in the 300–400 blood sugars turn it around and become a diet-controlled diabetic.

CONCLUSION

There will always be a new magical pill for your current diabetic crisis, but let me ask you this question, "If I have been implementing this diabetic diet to those patients of mine who want to participate and eliminate all those medications that they have to take every day to maintain their blood sugars, then why haven't they found the cure?" My statement is very simple: Just follow the money.

The answer is very clear. The cure is there. It is located between your two ears and starts with your mouth. There is a saying, "God gave you two ears and one mouth for a reason. Use them proportionally."

Are you willing to change your lifestyle and emotions, or are you going to keep your current crisis at your waistline? Are you going to listen to what is being presented to you, or are you going to start asking more questions? The choice is yours.

In my practice, when a patient truly applies this simple way of eating, it does not take long for their blood sugar number to drop. When the blood sugar starts dropping, the neuropathy symptoms of the tingling and burning sensations begin to reduce.

It is always my goal for my diabetic patients to have them all become diet-controlled and enjoy life. Once they can do this, then what? Turn the page and see the live-it lifestyle or the whole life diet for healthy people.

CHAPTER 11

The Holy Grail or the Holy Grill

The Live-It Lifestyle for the Whole Life Diet

––––––

We spend most of our time searching for the holy grail, but in actuality, it is on the *grill*—when we cook and what we cook. Thus, the term "holy grill" can be found in our home on the stove, the grill in our backyard, and even at the restaurant we eat at.

The greatest tragedy of life is that it takes a tragedy to change one's life!

Here is a simple pearl of wisdom: "It is not about dieting; it is about living!" Think about it. Our language is all about dying! Dead ends, deadlines, and die it (diet). Why not look for ways to live and incorporate it into a lifestyle? In some cases, we spend our whole life so worried about dying that we forget to live.

I have already explained some simple diets for the diabetic and low immune system, which were found in Chapter 9 and 10. In this chapter I will put together the whole life diet or what I would like to call live-it lifestyle. I encourage you to read through these pages, pick out what you can do today, and don't be overwhelmed by the material. In three or six months, you will set the course for the rest of your life. Welcome to how I see the world. I hope you will find the beauty just as I have found in living it through a lifestyle.

WHOLE LIFE DIET FOR THE BEST HEALTH AND LONGEVITY

The whole life diet is designed to live it. I call it a diet so I do not to leave you confused. Follow the whole life diet if you fall in the yin-yang scale between –3 and +3. That is the range where your immune system will really help you maintain a healthy way of life. The whole life diet is your key to healthy retirement planning. If you sidetrack, which happens at times, you may have to go back to the immune diet for a few days so you get back on course. I will also point out that knowing your blood type will help you in choosing which meats to eat.

When you approach this diet, in each category you will see multiple items to choose from. It is my recommendation to choose one thing that you want from each area on the list and do the daily recommended serving.

Here are the subheading for each category, and it is important to follow these as outlined. It is assumed when I mention anything in the important and good sections these items are organic, and those items in the avoid section contain GMO and GMF items.

- **IMPORTANT:** It's just that! It is important you follow and start implementing these food items into your daily regimen.
- **GOOD:** Does not have the quality as the important ones, but it does have the good qualities you will want to also

incorporate. It gives you more latitude for what to eat and drink.

- **POOR:** It's better than the avoid, but not as good as those items listed in the good section.
- **AVOID:** It's just that! Avoid at all measures. Avoiding these foods will help you transition to the whole life diet as most of the avoids in the whole life diet are also the same with a few variants.
- **COMMENTS:** This section will be listed at the bottom of each category and will give you greater insights.

I have simplified this diet because everyone is on a different level. This is only a quick reference guide. You can go to www. liveitlifestyles.com and print out a copy for yourself.

BEVERAGES, MINERALS, STIMULANTS, ALCOHOLS, AND TEAS

Important

- Water: Reverse osmosis (RO)
- ConcenTrace Minerals: 10–15 drops in some fluid (reverse osmosis water) or soups or other beverages
- Juices: Carrot, blueberry, cherry, unsweetened cranberry

Good

- Root Herb Teas: Rooibos, ginger
- Leaf Herb Teas: Raspberry, rooibos, cleavers, chamomile, burdock, yellow dock, dandelion, echinacea, ginseng

Avoid

- Stimulants: Caffeine, coffee, black and green teas, chocolate,

cocoa, cola drinks, energy drinks, NoDoz, Excedrin, cocaine, amphetamines
- Alcohol: Beer, wine, liquor
- Teas: Lipton, morning thunder, guarana mate, black mountain, earl grey, kali tea

Comments

- Mix ⅓ cup carrot juice with ⅓ cup RO water and ⅓ cup other vegetable juice. Drink a quart a day but only when you are feeling strong.
- It is best to have just a bit of color to the urine for proper hydration of the body and your cells.
- Watch your urine. If it has too much color all day, you will need to drink more, but if your urine is clear, drink less.
- Herb Tea Directions: Bring the water to a boil, put the herbs in. Simmer roots for 15 minutes or steep leaves for 3–5 minutes.

FERMENTED FOODS AND PROBIOTICS

Important

- Fermented Foods: Sauerkraut, yogurt, kefir, miso
- Seaweeds: Wakame, dulse, kelp, kombu nori, hijiki, agar, arame, bladderwrack, Irish moss, ogonori, mozuku

Good

- Probiotics: Acidophilus
- Fermented Foods: Organic soy foods such as miso, tempeh, natto

Avoid

- Soy Foods: Soy milk, soybean oil, soy flour, soy breads, edamame, tofu

Comments

- Take 2 capsules of acidophilus (probiotics) 2–4 times a day. Reduce to 1 time a day as you are doing better.
- Take the probiotics 30–45 minutes before a meal. This is so that it will be out of the stomach before the hydrochloric acid is produced by the stomach.
- A good brand of probiotics will have 5 billion active CFU/g that is found in the refrigerator section of the store.

OILS, REFINED OILS, AND FRIED FOODS

Important

- Oils: Krill oil, omega-3 oils, skate oil, salmon oil, cod liver oil, Organic Valley and Kerrygold butters

Good

- Oil: Olive, coconut

Avoid

- Oils: Canola oil, soybean oil, refined oils such as sesame and safflower, hydrogenated oils and heated oils, shortening, lard, oleo, margarine
- All oil vitamins such as A, D, E, and F, fish oils, omega-6 and omega-9 oils, flax oils, avocado oil
- Deep-Fried Foods: French fries, onion rings, nuts, corn chips,

potato chips, tempura, chicken, fish. Fatty food such as hamburgers, hot dogs, luncheon meats, sausage, bacon, butter

Comments

- Take 1–2 of the 350-mg capsules of krill oil 2 times a day. Costco has the best quality and least expensive called Kirkland krill oil.
- Omega-3 oils : Use at least 1–2 tablespoons each day using 100% grass-fed butter or fish liver oil.

FRUITS, VEGETABLES, SWEETS, AND SUGARS

- 2–4 servings a day. Fermented, salads, juice, soup, stew, stir-fry, steamed, casserole, or baked
- ¼–½ cup a day of fruits and berries
- 1–3 serving a day of 4–6 ounces of vegetable proteins

Important

- Dark Greens: Bok choy, dandelion, kale, collard, seaweed, beet, mustard, chard greens, spinach
- Stalk: Broccoli, celery, leeks, asparagus, green beans
- Root: Carrots, dandelion, burdock, onions, parsnips, rutabagas, turnips, radishes
- Salad Greens: Romaine, leaf, red, bib, arugula, spring mix, to name a few
- Spices: Cinnamon, cilantro, chives, ginger, garlic, oregano, thyme, basil, turmeric
- Salad Dressing: Mustard, lemon and lime juices, balsamic and apple cider vinegar; blend with any herbs
- Salts: Very good quality sea salt is important; tamari, miso
- Fermented: Sauerkraut and kimchi, cabbage, turnips, carrots, onions, cucumbers

- Seaweeds: Wakame, dulse, kelp, kombu, nori, hijiki, agar agar, aonori, ogonori, mozuku
- Berries
- Vegetable Proteins: Nuts, seeds, spirulina, bee pollen

Good

- Dark Green: Beets, mustard, chard, spinach
- Stalk: Brussels sprouts, cauliflower, cabbages
- Root: Beets
- Spices: Curry
- Fermented: Miso, tamari, tempeh, natto
- Fruits: Organic non-sweet ones such as stone fruits, apples, citrus, kiwis, pomegranates, watermelon, bananas, avocados, tomatoes
- Vegetable Proteins: Beans, legumes, lentils, peas, tempeh, natto

Avoid

- Stalk: Sweet corn (it will be GMO!)
- Vegetable Proteins: Soybeans and edamame and all GMO vegetable proteins

Comments

- Have ¼–½ cup of blueberries a day especially if cooked in oatmeal. Oatmeal with blueberries is best in the morning and can even be used as an evening treat.
- You may eat raw foods and vegetable juices only if you do not have phlegm, sinus or lung congestion, or you feel weak.

PROTEINS: ANIMALS

- Serve 4–6 ounces 4–7 times a week. Determine which types of animals to eat depending on blood type.

Important

- Chicken, wild fish, turkey, lean beef, lamb, pork, wild game, eggs, 100% grass-fed dairy products
- Wild-caught fish only, salmon

Good

- Wild-caught fish, tuna, shark, sea bass, marlin, halibut, swordfish, pike, walleye, shrimp

Avoid

- Farm-raised fish
- GMO grain-fed beef
- Caged chicken
- GMO, dairy products, milk, cheeses, cream, sour cream, ice cream, kefir, yogurt

Comments

- Have cilantro and fermented vegetables to detoxify the mercury that is found in the fish.
- Best to use animal foods for roasts, casseroles, soup and stew broth, or as a flavoring for dishes, sauces, and gravy

100% WHOLE GRAIN, REFINED GRAINS, SNACK FOODS, AND YEAST-CONTAINING FOODS

- 1–3 servings a day of cooked grains, cereals, casseroles

Important

- Organic brown rice, oatmeal, quinoa, spelt

Good

- Organic millet, barley, buckwheat, rye, toasted bread

Poor

- Corn, triticale, potatoes
- 100% whole wheat pasta, toasted bread

Avoid

- GMO soy and corn and all corn products unless labeled organic
- Refined Grains: White flour, unbleached flour, cracked wheat, most bread, pasta, pizza crust, pretzels, cereals, crackers
- 100% Whole Grain: All wheat flour products unless labeled whole wheat
- Snack Foods: Cakes, doughnuts, cookies
- Yeast-Containing Foods: Baking and nutritional brewer's yeasts and autolyzed yeast

Comments

- When making casseroles, cooked grains, or cereals, make sure to use organic ingredients.

- Eat only organic corn products; soy and corn are always GMO.
- If you have congestion, do not eat flour products such as wheat, buckwheat, rye, and corn triticale.
- Breads are good if you have no phlegm or congestion.

SAUCES, CHEMICALS, AND DRUGS
Avoid

- Sauces: Distilled vinegar, ketchup, most dressings and sauces like Worcestershire, Chinese plum, teriyaki, and sweet and sour, hot sauces, salsas, red curry, spaghetti sauce
- Drugs: All over-the-counter medications, especially Tylenol, NSAIDS (Ibuprofen, Motrin, Aleve, Advil, Tylenol, aspirin)
- Chemicals: Endocrine disrupters, steroids, antibiotics, HRT, HGH growth hormones
- Preservatives, flavor agents, MSG, glutamate, autolyzed yeast, casein, caseinate, commercial soup, broth, and sauces
- GMO and GMF genetically modified organisms or foods such as soy, corn, sugar beets, canola oil, and cotton seed oil

Comments

- Most sauces have MSG in them if they say hydrolyzed vegetable protein (HVP) or texturized vegetable protein (TVP)
- HRT, HGH growth hormones, steroids, and antibiotics are given to animals or put in milk; these are also known as endocrine disrupters and will have a very bad effect on the immune system and promote excessive cell growth.
- Avoid most vitamins and pills if called health products, as they are just chemicals and you do not need them.
- Generally, steamed foods are poor if you have a lot of phlegm.

SOY FOODS

Good

- Some fermented organic soy foods such as miso, tamari, tempeh, natto

Avoid

- All other soy foods: soymilk, soybean oil, soy flour and breads, edamame (raw soybeans in the pod)

GENERAL INFORMATION

- If you have phlegm, no raw foods or salads or cold beverages.
- Don't eat raw or cold foods. Do not have left over foods of more than a day old, as they may develop mold or bacteria in them.
- Avoid microwave devices especially at night, cell phones and remote phones, Wi-Fi, 5G, smart meters, and blue lights.
- Avoid overdoing things such as exercising, working, eating, worrying, thinking, and staying up too late at night.
- Avoid drafty rooms and getting chilled and cold feet. It is good to wear shoes and socks.
- To prevent getting chilled, dry your hair before going to bed so there is no wet hair on the neck or ears.
- Stay warm and dry. Get sunlight and movement.
- Read the labels of the things you buy. If you see words or names you cannot pronounce or recognize, you know it is not good for you.

EXERCISE

Exercise: Walk on a level surface at the beginning for fifteen minutes the first week and do this two times a day. Then increase by five minutes each week until you walk forty-five minutes a day. It is best to do this in a park where there are no man-made objects so your mind will not analyze things. Natural settings are more relaxing.

The best exercises: Walk, hike, stretch, dance, swim (backstroke). Yoga and tai chi are the best for longevity.

Do this daily but in moderate lengths so you aren't sore or drained the next day. Be consistent and build slowly.

It is best to exercise for twenty minutes a day as you get healthier, then build up to an hour per day. This will give the body mobility and strength over time.

CONCLUSION

The whole life diet is the balancer; it is the place you want to be. It is the bucket without the muddy water.

When you understand the yin-yang principles "hot and cold, weak and strong" and you apply the five elements and know your blood type along with the attitudes you presently have, this will give you a greater understanding for this way of life. As my Healthy Dad would say, living the "whole life diet" becomes your benchmark for eating healthy on a daily basis.

1. Enjoyable body movement is the key to physical health.
2. Grounding is the key to energy health.
3. Love is the key to true immunity.

REMEMBER: YOU CANNOT REMEDY A LIFESTYLE

Over time, you will transition to healthier foods, so take time to read the information presented. You will then learn more about what will improve your health. Work up to the improvements over the next few months, and in a year, you will transition to much healthier eating habits without a great struggle. Each month, reread this info and you will pick up on more things that you can easily improve. In other words, you cannot take a remedy and overcome a bad lifestyle. It takes a whole food diet, exercise, and rest to keep your biology in balance. Remedies, whether they are natural or are chemical drugs, will not enable you to be healthy if you do not take the steps to keep your body balanced. The general thing about food is to only have foods in their natural whole state with no chemicals added or unnatural processing done to the food, because it will change the simple natural balance of the food.

Avoid foods that are refined, preserved, genetically modified organisms or food (GMO/GMF), and ones that have chemicals added to them. Fast foods and snack foods have had processes done to them which remove the essential nutrients that are important to make the food more digestible and usable by the body. Keep your foods simple and whole, the way nature grew them, and you will not have to think about the individual nutrients.

Just know in nature when things are balanced, there is no disease!

Is there something that you could be doing today to bring your life more balance?

CHAPTER 12

Time Will Pass.
Will You?

———

In college, there was a clock that was positioned on the south wall of the biology lecture hall. I sat on the far-left side of the room so I could look over my right shoulder to see what time it was, as I had no cell phone, nor did I wear a watch. I only went by the clocks on the wall to determine if I was going to be late or early to the next class.

Under this clock, there was a sign that said, "Time will pass. Will you?" This was bothersome to me to the point that I would always look at the sign instead of paying attention to the professor. It's like that song you play on the way to work that you can't get out of your head for the rest of the day.

There are several principles that I applied from this saying on the wall.

First, in life there will be many distractions that will get you off course from your goals and aspirations. It is important to pay attention to what is in front of you at the present time, especially when it comes to what you are eating. If you know what you're eating and you protect your immune system, you can take the stress out of life when you eat healthy.

Second, fear hurts the kidney or inherent chi, and you only have so much of it. So protect it by staying out of future thoughts that cause you to stress over things. Personally, I don't stress about the flu or viruses that come and go every year. As long as I maintain my sound eating principles, I will be okay.

To have knowledge is freedom. In the early days of the biblical era when Adam and Eve were in the garden, they referred to the tree of life as good and evil. All Adam and Eve had to do was eat the fruit of the tree and they would have knowledge. Now, how cool is that? All you have to do is eat to have knowledge. Yes! But it must be the good quality of foods. It must be non-GMO and free from Roundup and chemicals.

We all have this tree of life within us. The better the quality of foods, water, and air we eat, drink, and breathe, the more freedom and knowledge we are able to receive. Back in Chapter 6, I spent a little time on the pineal gland. There was a reason for this: if you can keep yourselves free from the chemicals in your food and water and even the air that you breathe, you will have this untapped knowledge. It is given to everyone and I mean everyone—it is the empirical knowledge from a higher source.

THE THIRD LEADING CAUSE OF DEATH IN AMERICA IN 2013

An article from *Leapfrog Hospital Safety Grade,* published in Washington, DC on October 23, 2013, explains that hospitals are the third leading cause of death in the United States. New research estimates up to 440,000 Americans are dying annually from **preventable** hospital errors. The article goes on to say, "We are burying a population the size of Miami every year from medical errors that can be prevented."

It must also be pointed out that I did not mention heart disease and diabetes that kill thousands every year and could also be prevented.

In 2020, when the COVID-19 pandemic hit, the world deaths on December 31, 2020, by country, are recorded on the coronavirus website as follows:

COUNTRY	DEATH
United States	342,634
Brazil	193,875
India	148,738
Mexico	124,897
United Kingdom	72,657
Russia	56,271
Canada	15,523
China	4,634
Australia	909

The point I make here is this: the **preventable** hospital errors of 440,000 that ended in deaths just in America in 2013 is greater than deaths due to COVID in any of the above countries in the world, and yet there is very little public awareness on preventable death. Of those who passed away in 2013 from a hospital error, I wonder how many of them would still be alive if they had no reason in the first place to go to the hospital?

It is my opinion that the primary problem that makes the body more susceptible to viruses and illnesses such as COVID-19 is acidity level of the blood and a poor immune system. "When life is balanced, there are no diseases."

If this book could just make one person aware of their health and their current lifestyle and go to a more preventable way of living, the time and money spent in putting this book together was well worth it!

Since my interactions with my Healthy Dad, my approach to life has been all about prevention through a "live-it lifestyle" to stay healthy rather than a diet that is short-lived to stay healthy.

WHAT HAPPENS WHEN YOU DON'T LISTEN TO YOUR BODY?

It is said that experience is the best teacher. Sometimes these experiences are painful, some are rewarding, and some give you a different perspective on life. I would like to share with you one of those life experiences that was painful, but it led me to eventually finding my Healthy Dad many years later by asking many questions.

Back in Chapter 1, I introduced a brief anecdote about what I experienced while in medical school. I would like to go into greater detail, so some may be repetitive, but the experience I feel is important from the standpoint that life experiences become our greatest teacher, and when we ignore some of these painful experiences instead of trying to understand and learn from them, we miss the opportunity to learn at a higher level. I am hoping you will reflect back on some of those experiences in your life that need to be addressed and looked at as a teaching moment rather than a punishment.

While in medical school, I suffered from kidney stones all because I was not eating properly. Kidney stones come in different shapes and sizes. Mine at the time happened to be those little ones with spikes on them, and after my first episode in the fall of 1994 that landed me in the emergency room, I went to see a kidney specialist in San Francisco. He wanted me to get a study on my kidney to see if the stone had passed. It was a common procedure where they would inject a dye and the dye would light up on the X-ray if the stone was still present. The procedure was performed, and everything went well. I was given the green light that there were no remaining stones. I was never instructed on what I should eat or drink or what I should avoid. I was just told to drink lots of water. So I went back to my old eating habits. I ate to survive. You would think I would have learned from my first experience. It was not long when I had another kidney stone attack. It happened when I came home for a short visit to attend my brother's wedding in the early spring of 1995.

Feeling the pain in my right side again, at my Sick Dad's recommendation, I went to the local clinic to have it looked at. The primary doctor who actually introduced me to medicine examined me and sent me over to the hospital to get some tests run on me. I was once again offered the procedure to see if the stone was stuck in the kidneys.

The IV line was started and then the contrast dye was pushed into my body. This time, it was different. I had an awful taste in my mouth immediately. The lab tech had just gone back to take the first X-ray of the kidney, but she felt pressed to go back and check on me. It was a good call on her part as she witnessed that I had gone into a full-blown anaphylaxis reaction. I was having great difficulty breathing. For any of you who have experienced an anaphylaxis reaction, you can attest that it is much greater than a simple asthma attack.

The hospital code team was called in, and all the available medical personnel including the primary doctor who sent me to the hospital and the radiologist rushed in to provide medical attention to keep me alive. They started pumping medicine into my body to calm my heart rate, which was over 200. As I was still struggling to just get one breath in, my blood pressure dropped. It was when my blood pressure dropped that I stopped fighting to breathe on my own. It was there when I entered the most peaceful and beautiful place that I have ever experienced in my life. The lights that lit up the room were so pleasant that even today, when I try to paint them within my own artwork, the color always falls short of re-creating those brilliant bright lights. To me, it is something that did not exist on this earth. This place had no worries, fears, anger, or grief. I was not trying to do this or that. I was at complete peace and I wanted to stay. I could still see and hear the surroundings in the room, but I just couldn't speak. My thoughts were also present, and I recalled that I had made a promise to my brother that I would attend his wedding. That was when things changed, and I moved from this most beautiful place that I did not want to leave to a place of wanting to breathe again so I could fulfill my promise.

I later learned from what the doctor's report showed that the medical team spent three hours trying to resuscitate me. I was under the impression it was just minutes. During this time, the hospital personnel were notified to reach out to notify my father. Since my father only used a landline for talking on phones, the only way to find my father was to sound the local fire alarm that would send a message to all volunteer firefighters on their pager with a brief description regarding the fire. But this time there was no fire, only a message that was telling my uncle who was on the fire department that if he was anywhere near my father that he needed to get to the hospital as soon as possible. I later found out that my father, not knowing if he was going to the hospital to witness another son whom he would have to bury, went home, washed up, and put on some clean clothes and then went to the hospital.

I could only imagine what was going through his mind as I went through a similar experience with my daughter when I was given a similar notice by a phone call that my little girl had been stung by a bark scorpion and she developed a full-blown reaction and was headed to the emergency room when she was only two years old.

THE CHANGING POINT

Being in a place I did not want to leave, a thought was presented to me. It was the thought that I had made a promise to my brother to be at his wedding. My desire to stay in this place now shifted to "Can I just get one more breath to stay alive to fulfill that promise I made?" I was granted this breath, as I am here today to write about it. Once I regained consciousness, the first question I asked was, "Did someone turn on the lights in the room?" I find it amazing that I am always asking questions. "Always the student learning." As I had noticed when I first went into the X-ray room, the lights were on and I could easily see the surroundings of the room. The answer from the medical staff was, "No, there were no lights turned on." This led me to wonder what was this light that I had seen? The only way I can describe those lights is when I take someone into the operating room, there are two bright spotlights above the patient to help aid the surgeon to see the surgical area better. It was like these spotlights being turned on but even brighter and filling the entire room.

The part that will always remain with me from this experience is the feeling that I had while accompanied by the lights. It was that complete peace of mind as previously described. Anyone who has been there will say, "I did not want to come back."

My primary doctor made the comment to me when I came to, "Boy, you should not be here! Either you have a strong will to live, or you have some purpose in life to fulfill. You are very lucky."

My father arrived at the hospital to find me alive. I spent that night in the hospital for observation, and I did make it to my brother's wedding. "A promise made is a promise kept!"

I can tell you from my own personal experience, I was not tainted by medications that would alter my mind, such as morphine or painkillers. I experienced something that most only get to experience once, "that last drop of kidney chi or the last breath of life." I was given a second chance.

For those of you who have wondered what life is like on the other side, I can tell you that I have yet to find the colors that create the bright brilliant lights accompanied by the complete peace. The thing that separates our body from the spirit when we pass on is the inability to touch and to feel. The ability to touch and feel is only an earthly thing, but it's the one thing that I feel makes it so difficult for one who is on the verge of death to pass on, knowing that they will not have the ability to hug and kiss the ones they love again. You can see and hear, but those who have passed on want more than anything to have that ability to feel and touch again, from my personal opinion and experience.

I also feel strongly the reason why it was so difficult for everyone in 2020 with COVID-19 during the pandemic was the inability to give someone a hug and not being able to socialize with others. Human beings were always meant to be loving no matter what country, race, or family you come from. We were not meant to be isolated and alone. If laughter is the best medicine, then giving someone a hug is the best preventative medicine.

WHAT DID I OBSERVE FROM MY SICK DAD?

When you observe, you learn. You learn what to do and what not to do when you observe, but it is a power learning tool. While in my surgical residency program, there was a saying, "See one, do one, teach one." When you see one, you start to formulate the questions. When you do one, you apply what you observed and what you were taught, and then when you teach one, you incite someone else to ask the questions. This is why I say I will always be a student because I am always observing and formulating questions to learn from.

Here is what I observed from my Sick Dad. He was a good man. He had good intentions to help and serve those around him and even those he never met. I also observed this subtle thing: had my Sick Dad truly loved himself, I don't think he would have eaten the things he ate over the years that finally caught up to him. Was it his fault? No. Maybe he just did not know. I know we all have an expiration date when we are born, but that does not mean we stop living. Life is beautiful and meant to be lived to its fullest. By loving yourself, "God's greatest creation" (you), you can love others. That is why I refer to loving oneself in a humble way as the third greatest commandment.

I have mentioned many things in this book from the quality of foods we eat to reading what we eat, to the emotions, and how they affect us individually and differently. One thing I can tell you is that when we rush to the sugars and the sweets, we really need to do a self-evaluation and ask ourselves one important question: Do I enjoy who I am, or am I running from myself?

Our soul consists of the body and the spirit. In order to live, you need both. This requires good health, physically and mentally, eating real food according to your yin-yang constitution of that day, and having a good attitude that requires you to recognize one of the five elements of emotions that is part of you in some form or degree until you find that true and pure love that has no opposites. Is this possible? The answer is yes! We just need to be open to it.

MY SICK DAD ENTERED THE PLACE THAT I ONCE TRAVELED TO

A week prior to May 22, 2020, my Sick Dad asked me when I would be coming back home to see him. I had been wanting to go and see him, but with the state's shutdown orders, I postponed my trip, and I had to keep pushing out my date. I remember that during that call on May 16, I told him I would be there the following weekend. After wrapping up the clinic on Friday the 22nd, I set out to drive the nine-hour road trip back home. When I was only one hour into the trip, I got a phone call from my sister informing me that my father had just passed away.

I spent most of my time in the car reflecting on my Sick Dad. If he would have just listened to what I have been living for the past fifteen years, would he still be here? Had he just let things go and not taken life so seriously, would he still be here? When a person close to us passes on, we start to ask questions just as I did. We ask these what-if questions. I feel my Sick Dad still had so much to offer. I just wanted so much to ask him more questions and observe more of what he did.

I am so grateful for all the teaching that I learned from him when he allowed me to observe and get in a question here and there. I was also so grateful for the ability to prepare my Sick Dad for what he was about to step into, life after death. The last few months when his health was getting worse, I would talk about my near-death experience. I encouraged him to go to the lights when they are presented and to make sure to have no regrets when he left this life. Learn to find that peace on this earth. Anyone can have it, and you don't have to wait until you pass on to experience it. Leave the emotional trash of guilt, anger, sorrow, worry, and resentment on earth, and only take with you the true love that resides deep inside. If you fully understand that you are the light and that you are the full potential, take that and welcome that light when you depart. I strongly feel he did when he departed to the other side without any regrets or disappointments. He will be missed, but my memories of his teachings through observing him my entire life will continue to live on.

HOW HAVE I APPLIED BY WHAT I OBSERVED AND ASKING QUESTIONS?

How have I applied the principles of this book? I read all labels on everything I buy. I want to know what I am putting in my body. I take the daily detox nutrition mix every day. I listen to my body temperature when deciding on what to eat for that day. I also incorporate it into my practice for when a patient is willing to ask me a question regarding their health. I am ready to offer handouts to help them overcome diabetes, gout, or fungal infections by just changing how they eat. I strive to stay present each day. All the anger, worries, sorrow, fears, resentments I try to recognize and eliminate before they become so big that they will start to damage this body of mine. Being present is the best way and loving yourself so you can love others.

I encourage each of you to formulate your own questions each and every day. I once had a discussion with my youngest boy. He asked me, "What is the difference between heaven and hell?" I said to him, "Heaven is a place you get to ask all the questions you want; you can learn everything. Hell is a place you're not permitted to ask any questions, so you stop learning." His eyes got big and he said, "Dad, I want to go to heaven." I looked at him and said, "Son, you can have it right now; it's called heaven on earth! You don't have to wait to go to heaven to start asking your questions."

Life will give you experiences, painful or pleasant. You just have to be open to each experience so it can teach you something.

BECOMING THE TEACHER, WHAT QUESTIONS DO I HAVE FOR YOU?

It has taken me many years to get to where I am currently at. I am so excited that you made it this far in the book, but just because it is the last page of the book, it does not mean you're done, for it is only the beginning to your new and exciting world that you will create.

Below are some questions for you:

- Am I eating the proper fuels to give me the joy I dream of having once I retire?

- What can I do today to take personal responsibility for my health?
- Do I get sick easily?
- Am I medication-free?
- Do my joints ache and hurt?
- Did I look at the label on the food item that I just bought or that I consumed?
- Do I jump from diet to diet?
- If I am too yang, do I know how to get closer to balance?
- If I am too yin, do I know what will bring me closer to balance?
- When was the last time I exercised for more than thirty minutes?
- Can I retire healthy so I will be able to enjoy my wealth, or will it be used up in medical bills?
- What did I learn from this book that I can apply to my life immediately?
- Do I love myself enough to love others? Or do I gravitate toward temporary comfort foods to fill the space?
- If today was the last day on earth, could I honestly say within myself I am free of all the worries, sorrow, anger, fear, and resentments of life? Am I at peace with myself?
- Do I know who I am?

The key to your health starts with a question. If you don't have a question, then at least start observing your own health or the health of family members and friends. Don't judge them, but only educate yourself so the questions will start.

My final question to you is this: "Are you willing to participate in your own health?"

It is my wish that each of you will have a successful life, a life of joy and peace and comfort knowing that you can live out your days enjoying your life through eating to thrive! There is a question in all of us, and once you ask, the process to participate in your health begins. Behind every great invention, every creation, every idea that was put into action, and behind every painting or book written, was a question.

What started my journey with my Healthy Dad? I asked him this simple question: "Can you teach me what you just did to my daughter to allow her pain to go away so she can eat again?" Now over fifteen years later, I asked another question: "Do I have your permission to write a book on what you have taught me?"

Healthy Dad said, "Yes!" Now that this one is done, are you ready for the next one?

Acknowledgments

To my Healthy Dad who continues to answer my questions and is eager to share his profound knowledge.

To my Sick Dad, my father, who showed me by example that serving others is really what matters.

To my high school teachers and counselor, who thought I would never make it past high school.

To my wife, Xanthi, for her constant love and support and her angelic smile she freely gives me every day.

To my four children, you are the spark that lights my inner joy.

To my publishing company, Scribe Media, and all those who work there, for making this book possible.

To my patients whom I have had the honor to help and treat over the course of my twenty-one years in practice.

To you, the reader, who chose to take time out of your schedule to read some of the material in this book.

I SAY, THANK YOU!

About the Author

DR. GLEN N. ROBISON is a father, husband, podiatric surgeon, podiatric physician, artist, author, and a **student** who is always learning.

He specializes in natural foot cures from fungal toenails, to unstable ankles, diabetic feet, and more. He is a diplomate, American Board of Multiple Specialties in podiatry, board certified in primary care and podiatric medicine, is a Jin Shin Jyutsu practitioner and trained in the art of manipulation through myopractics.

He has been personally applying the principles found in this book for over fifteen years while sharing it with thousands of patients.

He is medication-free and cannot recall the last time he has been seen by a doctor with the one exception being when he looks at himself in the mirror. LOL!

He was one of two surgeons who served a medical mission to the Kingdom of Tonga in August 2000.

He lectures on the base knowledge found in this book to group settings.

Outside his podiatric medical practice, he enjoys realistic oil painting and being in the outdoors. He resides in Arizona with his beautiful wife.

www.liveitlifestyles.com

Made in the USA
Las Vegas, NV
18 June 2021

24980978R00152